KAMA SUTRA NIGHTS

Quarto.com

© 2025 Quarto Publishing Group USA Inc.

First Published in 2025 by Fair Winds Press, an imprint of The Quarto Group,
100 Cummings Center, Suite 265-D, Beverly, MA 01915, USA.
T (978) 282-9590 F (978) 283-2742

All rights reserved. No part of this book may be reproduced in any form without written permission of the copyright owners. All images in this book have been reproduced with the knowledge and prior consent of the artists concerned, and no responsibility is accepted by producer, publisher, or printer for any infringement of copyright or otherwise, arising from the contents of this publication. Every effort has been made to ensure that credits accurately comply with information supplied. We apologize for any inaccuracies that may have occurred and will resolve inaccurate or missing information in a subsequent reprinting of the book.

Fair Winds Press titles are also available at discount for retail, wholesale, promotional, and bulk purchase. For details, contact the Special Sales Manager by email at specialsales@quarto.com or by mail at The Quarto Group, Attn: Special Sales Manager, 100 Cummings Center, Suite 265-D, Beverly, MA 01915, USA.

29 28 27 26 25   1 2 3 4 5

ISBN: 978-0-7603-9638-4

Digital edition published in 2025
eISBN: 978-0-7603-9639-1

Library of Congress Cataloging-in-Publication Data available.

Design and Page Layout: Quarante Douze Studio: Emmanuelle Desfossés & Antoine Foisy
www.quarantedouze.ca
Cover and Illustration: Mark-Antoine Thibodeau Breault

Printed in Hong Kong

The information in this book is for educational purposes only. Any type of sexual activity should be consensual.

QUIVER

KAMA SUTRA NIGHTS

64 Classic Sexual Positions for Couples of All Kinds

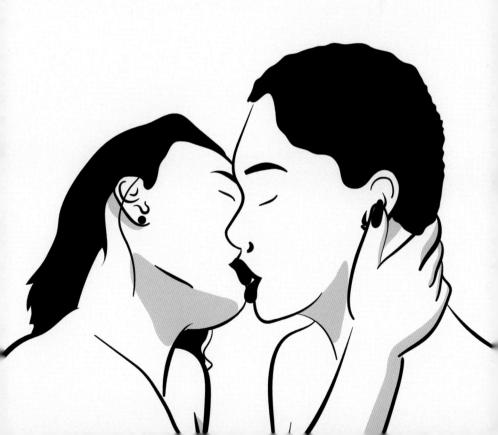

Contents

Introduction	7
A Note on Terms in This Book	11
How to Use This Book	12

The Positions

1	Nominal Kissing	16	20	The Monkey	55
2	Wrestling of the Tongues	17	21	The Union of Fixing a Nail	56
3	Pressing Yoni Kiss	18	22	The Union of the Spinning Top	59
4	Kissing the Yoni Blossom	21	23	The Union like a Swing	60
5	Sucking a Mango Fruit	22	24	The Turning Union with Giver on Top	63
6	Consuming the Lingam	25	25	The Full-Pressed Union	64
7	The Kiss of the Crow	28	26	The Half-Pressed Union	67
8	The Kiss of the Crow—Variation	31	27	The Packed Union	68
9	The Splitting of the Bamboo	32	28	The Yawning Position	71
10	The Bud	35	29	The Yawning Position—Variation	72
11	The Outstretched Clasping Position	36	30	The Widely Opened Position	75
12	The Side-by-Side Clasping Position	39	31	The Wife of Indra	76
13	The Conch	40	32	The Amazon	79
14	The Union like a Crab	43	33	The Feet Yoke	80
15	The Churning of the Cream	44	34	The Knot of Fame	83
16	The Flag of Cupid	47	35	The Lotus	84
17	The Flower in Bloom	48	36	The Peacock	87
18	Indrani	51	37	The Swing	88
19	The Lotus-like Position	52	38	The Trapeze	91

39 The Union like a Pair of Tongs	92
40 The Tortoise	95
41 The Peddling Tortoise	96
42 The Yab Yum Position	99
43 The Ass	100
44 The Cat	103
45 The Congress of the Cow	104
46 The Rutting of the Deer	107
47 The Dog	108
48 The Pressing of the Elephant	111
49 The Congress of the Elephant	112
50 Inversion	115
51 One Knot	116
52 The Rhino	119
53 The Rear-Entry Stride	120
54 The Thunderbolt or the Wheelbarrow	123
55 The Wrestler	124
56 The Encircling	127

57 The Face-to-Face Position	128
58 Fame	131
59 The Knee-Elbow Position	132
60 Two Palms	135
61 The Standing Stride	136
62 The Suspended Position	139
63 The Standing Swing	140
64 The Tripod	143

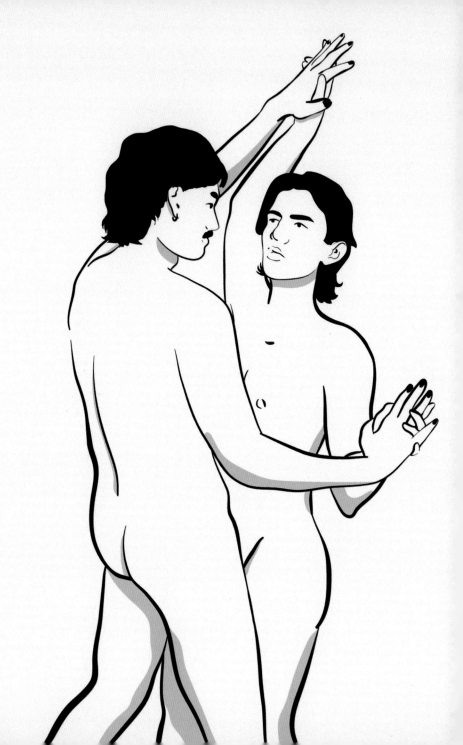

Introduction

Most people think of the Kama Sutra as a book full of bendy sex positions, but it's much more than that. The ancient Indian Hindu Sanskrit text is a lifestyle manual that covers issues great and small, including how to start and maintain a relationship, techniques for personal grooming, how to treat your friend's wife, and even the proper way to have an affair (send a messenger to get things going, FWIW).

But you're probably not here for the stuff like how to master the sixty-four arts (number forty-one is "the art of cock fighting, quail fighting, and ram fighting," if you want to get on that). You are here for the sex stuff, and fear not, you'll get your sex positions. Many of them are indeed excessively bendy, so do your stretching.

But the Kama Sutra has lots more to say about sex than how to put Body Part A into Body Part B. The text offers detailed instructions on various ways to kiss, different oral sex techniques, and ways to thrust and grind against each other. It also offers advice on what to do when partners have different speeds of arousal or unequal levels of passion.

The Kama Sutra not only describes how to do certain moves but the proper occasions for when to bust them out. For example, one of the kisses is "a kiss that awakens," which is when "a lover coming home late at night kisses his beloved, who is asleep on her bed in order to show her his desire. On such an occasion the woman may pretend to be asleep at the time of her lover's arrival, so that she may know his intention and obtain respect from him." I know many among us have done just that.

The Kama Sutra likes to get *extremely* specific with its categorizations of love, courtship, and sex. A "demonstrative kiss," for example, is "when at night at a theatre, or in an assembly of caste men, a man coming up to a woman kisses a finger of her hand if she be standing, or a toe of her foot if she be sitting, or when a woman is shampooing her lover's body, places her face on his thigh (as if she were sleepy) so as to inflame his passion, and kisses his thigh or great toe." If that exact situation comes up, you know what to do.

Types of Kissing

The Kama Sutra takes kissing *seriously*.

Nominal: Let only your lips touch.

Throbbing: When your lips touch, "pulse" your bottom lip.

Touching: Touch your partner's lips with your tongue like a snake, while closing your eyes.

Straight: A nominal kiss with your bodies and lips facing straight toward each other.

Bent: A deep-locking kiss with your tongues penetrating fully and your hands cupping each other's necks.

Turned: Put your hands on your partner's face to tilt it up then kiss them slowly and with passion.

Pressed: Hold your partner's lower lip, gently touch their lip with your tongue, then kiss them fully.

Upper lip: Suck the upper lip of your partner while they suck your lower lip.

Clasping: Take your partner's lips into your own, adding your tongue as you please.

Fighting of the tongues: Wrestle with each other's tongues and touch your tongues to each other's teeth, gums, and palates.

There's also info on a bunch of different types of scratches and nail markings and when to do them, intentions and techniques for biting one another, and various ways to strike each other. Some of that advice is sprinkled throughout these positions if you want to test out some BDSM practiced circa the second to third century CE.

Some of these positions look similar to each other, but there are subtle differences that give each its own unique vibe. Some of them use a grinding or churning rather than a thrusting motion; others are dependent on the receiver squeezing the muscles of their yoni (vagina) around a lingam (penis) or lingam equivalent to enhance both of your pleasure. Others are playful, rough, or silly and are mainly just about vibes.

If you want to go full-on authentic, here's a quick Kama Sutra vocab lesson.

Lingam	Penis
Yoni	Vulva, uterus, and/or vagina
Flowering lotus	The outer vulva, including the clitoris
Congress	Having sex

Is the Kama Sutra Still Relevant Today?

Yes and no. Some of it is spot-on all these eons later. Behold this wisdom on how to tell if someone with a vulva is satisfied or not:

"The signs of the enjoyment and satisfaction of the woman are as follows: her body relaxes, she closes her eyes, she puts aside all bashfulness, and shows increased willingness to unite the two organs as closely together as possible. On the other hand, the signs of her want of enjoyment and of failing to be satisfied are as follows: she shakes her hands, she does not let the man get up, feels dejected, bites the man, kicks him, and continues to go on moving after the man has finished."

People with vulvas can confirm: This still basically tracks.

Other parts are blunt and insightful about human desire. The section on "types of congress" acknowledges that thinking about someone else during sex is—okay, *fine*—a Thing We Do. "When a man, from the beginning to the end of the congress, though having connection with the woman, thinks all the time that he is enjoying another one whom he loves, it is called the 'congress of transferred love.'"

But other stuff is not so useful or even particularly relatable. There is no need to know that the Kama Sutra reports that women in a certain region "are fond of foul pleasures, and have not good manners." #Rude and #MaybeRacist. We also won't report on the love potion to bewitch someone using "a powder made of wind-blown leaves, flowers left on a corpse, and peacock bones." Though, if you have some peacock bones handy, no one needs to know what you do with them.

In the same way, not all these sex positions are going to be relevant to you. Some are going to be sexy and useful; others will be more like "go get some corpse flowers" and probably work better on paper. Some require a fuckton of flexibility and look like something human bodies—or at least your human body—aren't supposed to do. That's cool—be not ashamed! If you try something and it makes you feel like returning to the safety of missionary, go right ahead. BUT other positions are going to be hot—super hot—and are gonna give you a launching point to a shinier, happier sex life. You get to figure out which is which.

A Note on Terms in This Book

Even though the Kama Sutra is surprisingly woke about sexuality and talks about a third gender—"women acting as men"—and goes a little kinky with all the hitting, scratching, and biting, it uses the terms "man" and "woman." To modernize the text and make it more inclusive, we're using the term "receiver" for anyone getting penetrated by a penis or strap-on. The "giver" is the owner of said penetrating penis or strap-on. For positions involving oral sex, it's sort of the opposite: The giver is the one sucking, licking, kissing, or otherwise ravishing their partner's yoni or lingam. The receiver is one the being ravished. Yes, it's kind of complicated, but we can do hard things!

The book uses nongendered language and is written so you can switch these positions up with whatever y'all have going on gender- and sexuality-wise. The exceptions are the oral sex positions that focus exclusively on how to best love up a vulva or penis. If there's not a penis in the house (store bought or biological), no one's going to be giving a blow job. Just turn a few pages to the cunnilingus part and you'll be just fine.

How to Use This Book

Use these sixty-four sex positions however you'd like: vacation sex inspiration, items for your sex bucket list, or just what's gonna be happening next Thursday. Use and abuse it as you please. Go through it with your partner and mark which ones you'd both like to try. Take turns suggesting a position, then give it a go. Pick a standing, sitting, and lying down position and work them into a single session. Try them all, or try just the ones that don't look too bendy. Your body, your choice.

If a position requires some flexibility that you're not feeling, that's totally fine. Not everyone can bend their limbs into the lotus position. Go ahead and skip that one, wait until you've hit more yoga classes, or change it so it does work for you.

Feel free to tweak the positions in the book to fit you. Queer 'em up, have the straightest sex ever—it all works. You can add strap-on play, use different holes, fire up some toys, or add whatever else does it for you.

And if you want to get a little kinky, the Kama Sutra says it's A-OK. It goes hard with talk about hitting, biting, and scratching during sex. It even lists the eight types of nail marks you can leave on your lover's skin (for the record, they're discus, half-moon, circle, line, tiger's claw, peacock's foot, hare's leap, and lotus leaf). So hit, bite, and scratch away—with enthusiastic consent, of course.

TL;DR: Figure out whatever is going to make your yoni/lingam happy—then do that.

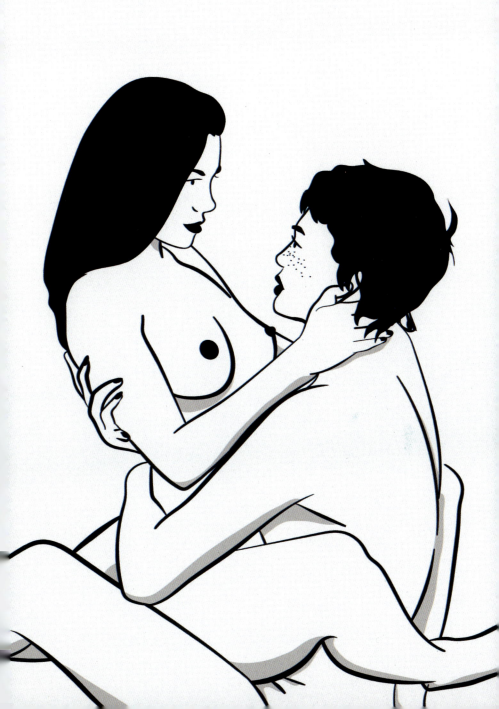

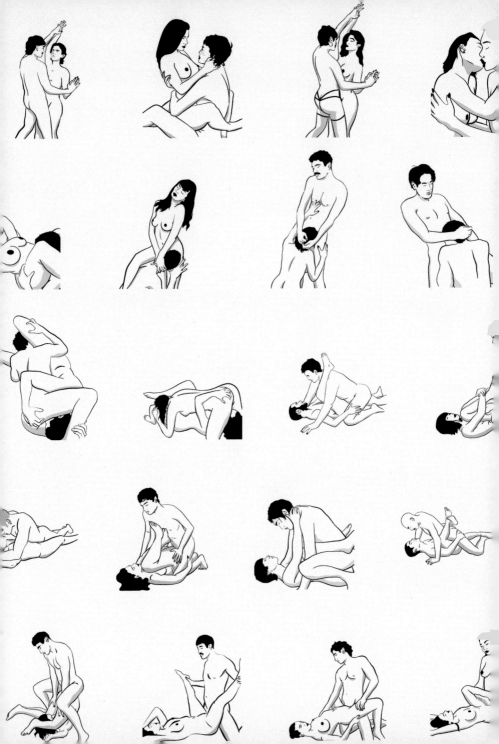

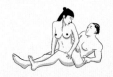

The Positions

1 Nominal Kissing

Just a little kiss.

How to Do It

In the Kama Sutra, nominal kissing is simply letting your lips touch. Just lean in and touch your lips together gently.

What's Good About It

This is a simple "how you doin'?" kind of kiss to start exploring each other and begin to breathe each other in. Kissing is an intimate way to access your partner's scent, taste, and feel and get a preview of how they will treat sex. Are they rushed or attentive? Do you like how they feel against your mouth? Do you want more or less? These are clues! Use them.

Tweak It

Breathe in unison while *just* touching your lips to connect and bring yourselves into the moment together. If you're feeling brave (or creepy), try the kiss with your eyes open.

Make It Even Better

The Kama Sutra is big on categorizing stuff and lists several kinds of kisses. You can add a "throbbing" kiss, which is pulsing the bottom lip when the lips touch or a "touching" kiss when you dart your tongue out like a snake and touch your lover's lips. Or try the "upper lip," which is sucking the upper lip of your partner while your lower lip is sucked.

2

Wrestling of the Tongues

Go off-label.

How to Do It

Wrestling of the tongues takes nominal kissing even further—to every place on your bodies. Want to kiss a part of your partner's body? Do that. Find another part. Kiss it. Repeat, repeat, repeat.

What's Good About It

Kissing is a sexy and intimate way to explore your partner's body, build arousal, and show affection and passion for each other.

Tweak It

Explore your partner's entire body with a series of kisses. Instead of going straight for the mouth-boobs-groin trifecta, linger on less obvious spots such as the eyelids, earlobes, back of the knee, arch of the foot, belly, inner arm, and/or the nape of the neck. Before you kiss a spot, hover over it a moment with your mouth and let them just feel your warm breath.

Make It Even Better

The Kama Sutra categorizes four styles of kissing and what body parts they are for. Try the "soft kiss," using gentle nips and licking on chests and various crevices. The "moderate kiss" is nibbling with teeth and used on the cheeks, breasts, hips, and belly. The "full-on kiss" is kissing the whole body and licking your partner's curves. And the "contracted kiss" is adding scratching to your partner's lips and body, which IDK, maybe?

THE POSITIONS

3 Pressing Yoni Kiss

Get some of that lotus power.

How to Do It

The receiver lies on the edge of the bed with their legs spread. The giver kneels on the floor with their head between their partner's legs. The giver presses their mouth into their partner's vulva, as though they're kissing them.

What's Good About It

This is a beginning move to warm up the receiver, and it shows respect for the receiver and their body (mainly their vulva, but still.) The giver doesn't even go in too deep, just kisses the vulva with no tongue.

Tweak It

The giver can go slowly to build their partner's arousal. Before starting they can place their open mouth next to the vulva and gently exhale warm breath. As they kiss, they can use their hands to rub and stroke their partner's belly, thighs, and boobs.

Make It Even Better

In eastern cultures, women and their yonis (a.k.a. vulvas, a.k.a. lotus flowers) are respected for being the givers of life. It is believed that stimulation of the vulva releases sexual energy, which flows out in juices. If you drink these juices, you fill yourself with sexual energy and power. Even if you don't necessarily believe that, if you act as though it's true, it's gonna be one fine oral session.

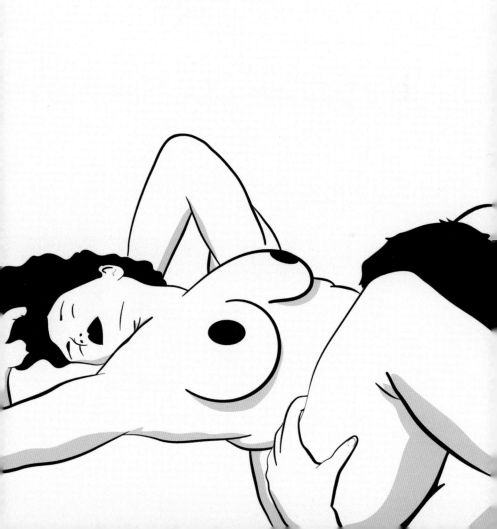

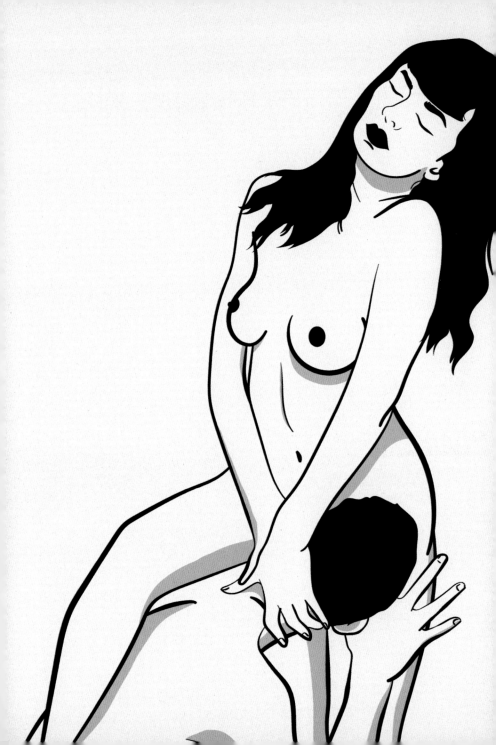

4

Kissing the Yoni Blossom

We're going in.

How to Do It

The receiver stands with their legs apart. The giver kneels in front of them between their legs and spreads their outer labia (the fleshy part of the vulva) apart, holding them open. (If standing is not your jam, the receiver can sit or lie down on something comfortable.) The giver licks up the shaft of the clitoris, running their tongue up each side, then adding long, slow sucks.

What's Good About It

Um, "long slow sucks."

Tweak It

The Kama Sutra recommends that you start with soft and shallow flicking licks along the shaft of the clit, then move to gently sucking on the clitoris and caressing it with your tongue. If the giver does lots of that, they'll be pretty golden.

Make It Even Better

Try for squirting with "the kiss of the penetrating tongue" where the giver thrusts their tongue inside of the vagina, then slides it back out, repeating and increasing speed as their partner gets closer to orgasm. For a more intense sensation, the giver can also focus their tongue on the clit and vulva and slide a finger or two inside the vagina, pressing on the upper wall. Keep doing this, then take cover.

THE POSITIONS

5

Sucking a Mango Fruit

Suck my fruit.

How to Do It

The receiver sits on a chair, stands, or lies down face up with their hips at the edge of the bed. The giver kneels between their partner's legs to take their lingam (a.k.a. penis) into their mouth. The giver takes their partner's penis halfway into their mouth, using lots of suction—like sucking on a lollipop or—as the name says—a ripe mango.

What's Good About It

A really great blow job is hot for both people. For the giver, it's a heady (. . .) experience to completely control someone's arousal and watch them respond to every lick, suck, and kiss. And the receiver gets to experience the glories of someone fully attending to them and one of their favorite body parts.

Tweak It

Eye contact and stroking the giver's hair is a great way for the receiver to signal how much they're into it or what more (or less) they might want. Plus they get the eternally enjoyable sight of watching someone take their lingam into their mouth.

Make It Even Better

Try the "side nibbling lingam kiss." The giver holds the penis with their fingers and kisses and nibbles in a gentle manner up and down each side of the shaft.

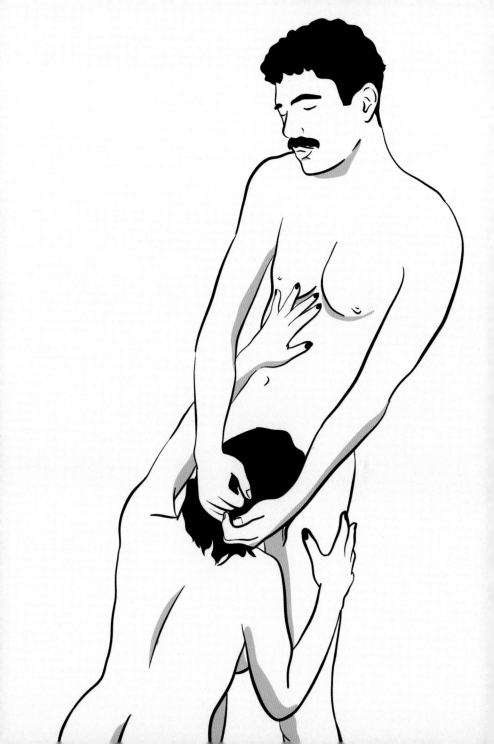

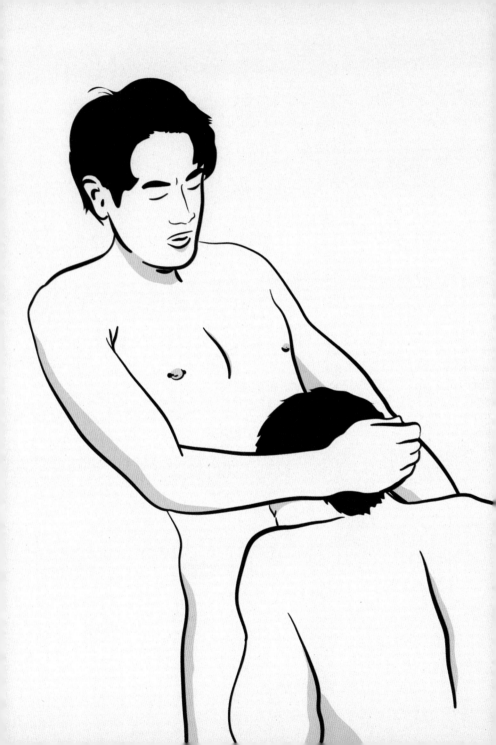

6 Consuming the Lingam

Basically, Kama Sutra for "deep throat."

How to Do It

Get in a position that's comfortable for both of you—either lying down, standing plus kneeling with the receiver bracing themselves against a wall, or sitting with the giver kneeling on the floor. The giver takes their partner into their mouth and slides it as far back into their throat as feels comfortable. If there's gagging, that's normal. Some people are turned on by it, some aren't. Do what works for you.

What's Good About It

The receiver gets the feeling of their penis being fully enveloped in warm wetness.

Tweak It

To make deep throating easier, the giver can open the back of their throat by pretending to yawn. Breathe slowly and easily through your nose, taking the penis in slowly. And if deep throating is really not the giver's jam, they can either stop and switch to a regular old BJ (totally fine!) or make it a semi-deep throat, wrapping their lubed-up hand around the base of the penis to mimic the feel, but with 100 percent less gagginess.

Make It Even Better

To get that lingam in as deeply as possible, the giver can lie on a bed with their head hanging back over the edge. The receiver stands at the side and the giver pulls them in as deep as they'd like by holding their hands on their butt cheeks.

The Kama Sutra Oral Quick Reference Guide

In case the last eight pages was too much reading.

What to Do If You Have a Vulva in Front of Your Mouth

Outer Yoni Tongue Strokes

Gently open your partner's labia (outer and inner lips) while gently kissing, licking, and probing with your tongue.

Inner Yoni Tongue Strokes

Open your partner's outer labia and lick their inner lips.

Flutter of the Butterfly

Kiss your partner's vulva while softly fluttering your tongue along the shaft of their clitoris.

Kissing the Yoni Blossom

Lick the clitoris on either side of their shaft, run your tongue across the head, and give long, sensual sucks to your partner's vulva. See page 21 for more details.

Sucking the Yoni Blossom

Tenderly suck your partner's clitoris in a gentle, tender manner, caressing their clitoris with your tongue.

Kiss of the Penetrating Tongue

Begin with shallow, flicking licks of your partner's vagina entrance. Penetrate and withdraw your tongue, increasing pressure. As their excitement increases, thrust your tongue deeper.

Drinking from the Fountain of Life

Relish and drink in the juices of sex, celebrating sexual energy as well as the energy of life.

What to Do If You Have a Penis in Front of Your Mouth

Nominal Lingam Kiss

Hold your partner's penis in your hand and place your lips around it, moving their penis in your mouth. Use your lips to press and release, pulling your mouth away.

Side Nibbling Lingam

Hold your partner's penis in your fingers and kiss and nibble in a gentle manner up and down the sides.

Outside Pressing Lingam Kiss

Gently press the head of your partner's penis, kissing it gently while sucking it like a straw.

Inside Pressing Lingam

Put your partner's penis into your mouth, keeping your lips firm and sucking with great force, then slowly withdraw their penis from your mouth.

Sucking a Mango

Take your partner's penis halfway into your mouth and suck with intense pressure.

Kiss the Lingam

Hold your partner's penis firmly in your hand while kissing the head and pressing and moving your lips gently.

Lingam Tongue

Stroke your partner's penis with your hand while licking and stroking with your tongue.

Consuming the Lingam

Take your partner's penis deep into your mouth and throat.

7

The Kiss of the Crow

The 69 of yore.

How to Do It

Both of you lie on the bed on your sides and facing each other with your faces between each other's legs for mutual oral sex. You can do one person on top and the other on the bottom, or try both of you lying on your sides.

What's Good About It

When you're giving and getting, you can mirror each other's actions and excitement level to create an intimate shared experience.

Tweak It

Use your tongue, fingers, and lips to mix up the stimulation. Don't worry about it being "equal" every second. One person is totally allowed to slack off a bit and just enjoy the sensations while the other focuses on them. This is especially helpful if the simultaneous giving and getting is overwhelming or when one of you is slower to get turned on. Trade back and forth, go at the same pace—up to you.

Make It Even Better

The Kama Sutra didn't mention sexy toys specifically, buuut if you want to use sex toys to amp up your pleasure, go ahead and fire some up. You can add butt plugs (vibrating or not); bullet, wand or clitoral suction vibrators; prostate vibrators; penis sleeves—whatever y'all have in your secret sex toy drawer.

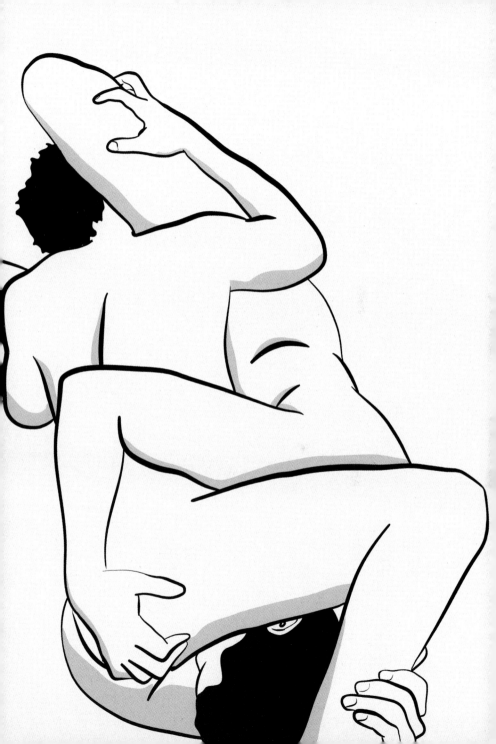

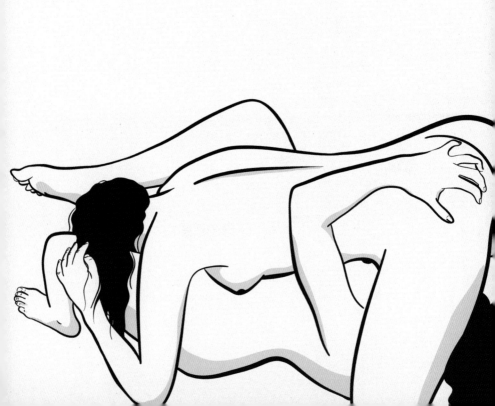

8

The Kiss of the Crow—Variation

No actual crows involved.

How to Do It

One person lies on the bed with their legs spread and their head hanging over the side. The other person stands by the partner's head and leans over to put their penis or vulva in their partner's mouth and put their own mouth between their partner's legs.

What's Good About It

This version of 69 lets you both comfortably enjoy the taste of your partner while their mouth and hands work on you at the same time.

Tweak It

If the person standing is feeling strong, they can lift their partner's hips and lick and nibble their partner's thighs and/or press their penis or vulva more firmly against their mouth.

Make It Even Better

Use your hands to enhance the actions of your mouth. Hold onto each other's butt cheeks to squeeze or pull each other closer. Slide a finger inside a vagina to rub the upper wall. Circle a wet thumb and forefinger around the base of the penis shaft. Give love to a set of balls with gentle sucking, long licks, or just cupping them with a hand. Slide a lubed finger in each other's asses. Listen to each other's moans to figure out what's working.

9

The Splitting of the Bamboo

Put your right foot in, put your right foot out.

How to Do It

The receiver lies on their back with their legs bent. The giver kneels by their partner's hips, puts one hand on either side of their head, and leans over their body. The receiver raises one leg and places it over their partner's shoulder, then straightens their other leg along the back. The giver straightens the same leg as their partner's on the same side (i.e., giver's left, receiver's right). The giver's tucked leg is the same one that the receiver has over their shoulder (i.e., giver's right, receiver's left).

What's Good About It

This is a good way to tart up regular ol' missionary.

Tweak It

Whether you decide to go in anally or vaginally, this position works for deep or shallow penetration—also a perk if you're working with an extra large or extra small penis or strap-on. For deeper penetration, the receiver pulls their raised knee back further; for more shallow penetration, the receiver pushes back with their leg against the giver's chest.

Make It Even Better

Try switching legs during it. It keeps everyone from getting sore, plus during the transition, the receiver can squeeze their vaginal or anal muscles around the penis or strap-on.

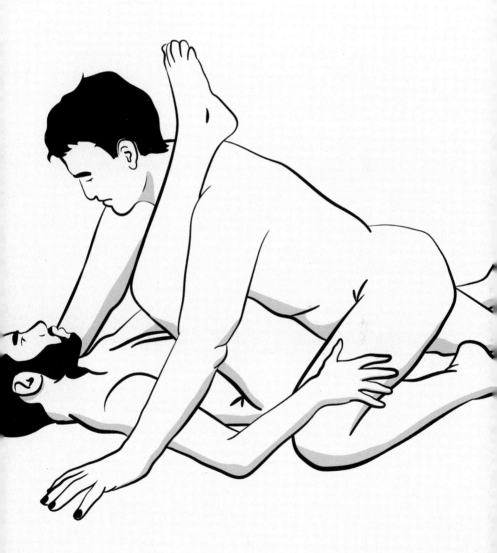

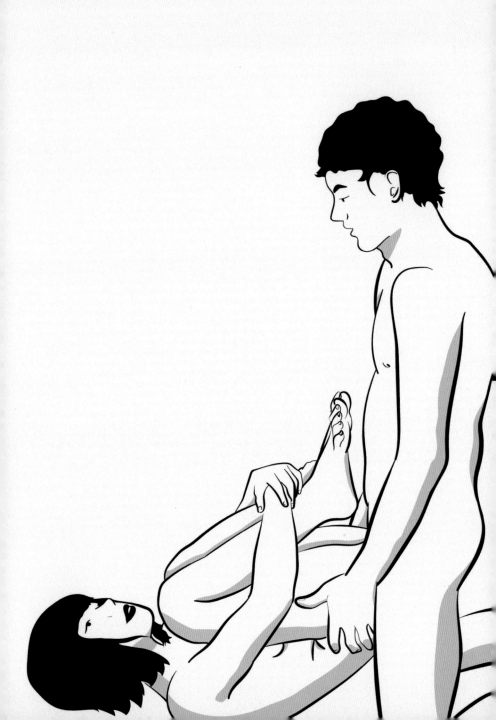

10

The Bud

Curl up and sigh.

How to Do It

The receiver lies on their back, tucking their knees up to their chest—kind of like they're rolled up into the fetal position. They can hold their knees in place with their arms or hands for more support. The giver kneels by their partner's bum to penetrate.

What's Good About It

Extremely deep penetration, whether you're going in anally or vaginally. (If it's too much penetration, the receiver can press their feet against their partner's chest to help guide how deep it goes.)

Tweak It

Put a sex wedge or a firm pillow or two under the receiver's hips for comfort and to get body parts exactly where you want them to go. The receiver can also rock their hips up and down to switch up the stimulation for both partners.

Make It Even Better

The Kama Sutra lists several ways of thrusting, and The Bud works well with the churning method. The giver holds their penis or strap-on in their hand and swirls it inside their partner's anus or vagina. If the receiver has a vulva, the giver can also pull out occasionally and swirl their head in a circle around their partner's clit.

11 The Outstretched Clasping Position

Hey, you.

How to Do It

The receiver lies flat on their back with their legs straight and slightly spread. The giver lies flat on top of their partner so they're completely covering their body, then stretches their legs straight between their partner's. Both people stretch their arms over their heads so they can hold hands.

What's Good About It

Lots of skin-to-skin contact, kissing, soulful eye contact, and hand holding during fuckery. So romantic!

Tweak It

If the person on the bottom has a vulva, the top person can shift their body up slightly so their partner can get more clit stimulation by pressing against their pubic bone. If a penis or strap-on is involved, the person on top moves up enough so that the top of their penis or strap-on is rubbing over the clit. Instead of thrusting, use more of a rocking or grinding motion, letting the bottom person guide the speed, motion, and pressure.

Make It Even Better

Throw down some old sheets or towels, cover yourselves in an excessive amount of lube or massage oil, and slide your bodies together. Then, for a tighter feel with penetrative sex, the receiver moves their legs between their partner's and presses them tightly together.

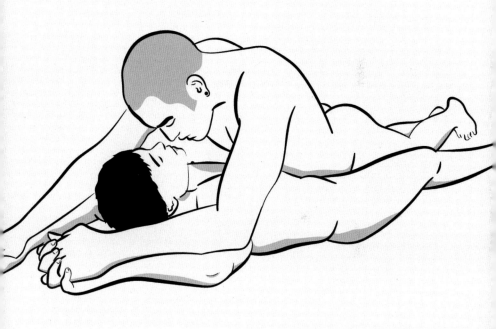

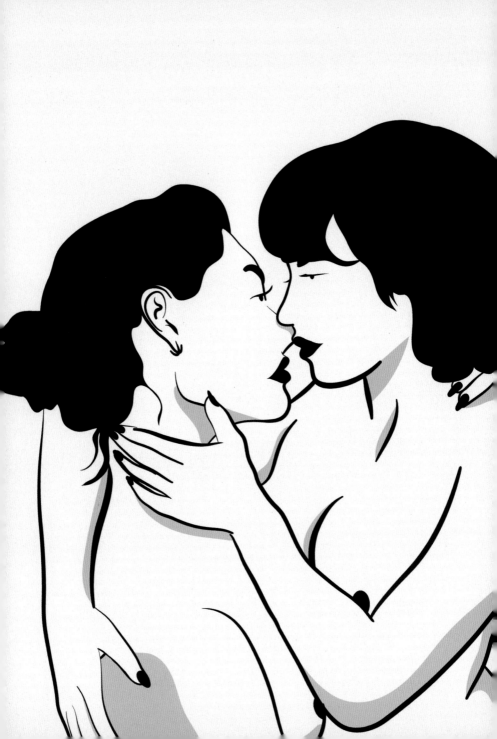

12 The Side-by-Side Clasping Position

So swoony.

How to Do It

Both people lie on their sides facing each other. Wrap your arms and legs around each other, pulling yourselves even closer.

What's Good About It

This is good for sleepy wake-up sex, slow and intense date night sex, and lazy weekend sex when you're spending all day in bed together. With all the intimate eye contact, opportunities for long slow kisses, and skin-to-skin contact, this is pretty much the most romantic position allowed by law.

Tweak It

Some people get turned on quickly, some more slowly. Some people feel completely done after an orgasm, some are still aroused afterward and want more touch. The Kama Sutra noted the differences in how people experience arousal and advised that people with similar arousal styles generally have better sexual compatibility, but work with what you've got. Make sure both of you get the time you need to be fully aroused and figure out a post-orgasm ritual that leaves you both well satisfied.

Make It Even Better

Add some more directed stimulation by slipping your hands or a toy or two down between your bodies. It makes everything better in both penetrative and nonpenetrative versions of this.

13

The Conch

Who knew squatting could be so sexy?

How to Do It

The receiver lies on their back and brings their knees up to their chest. The giver squats by their partner's butt and leans over their partner's body, resting their weight on their hands. The giver puts their thighs outside their partner's and presses together tightly.

What's Good About It

Because the giver is pressing their thighs together, it makes for a tighter feel for both partners. This position also situates a penis or strap-on so it's pointing more upward for delightfully targeted rubbing against a G-spot or P-spot.

Tweak It

The receiver has their hands free to stroke themselves or hold onto a small toy.

Make It Even Better

For better support and movement, plus even more targeted internal stimulation for the receiver, the giver can hold up their partner by the hips or butt. Or go ahead and let a pillow or two do the work. Use a specially designed sex pillow, or you can DIY it with regular pillows, sofa cushions, or even bunched-up sheets or towels. Be generous with the cushioning—pillows can also provide comfy support to necks, shoulders, and arms.

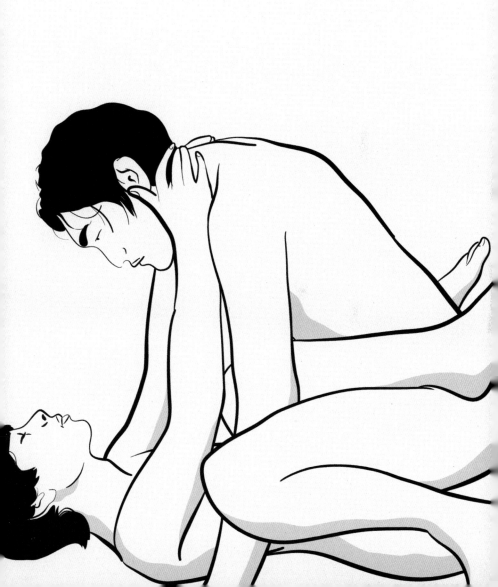

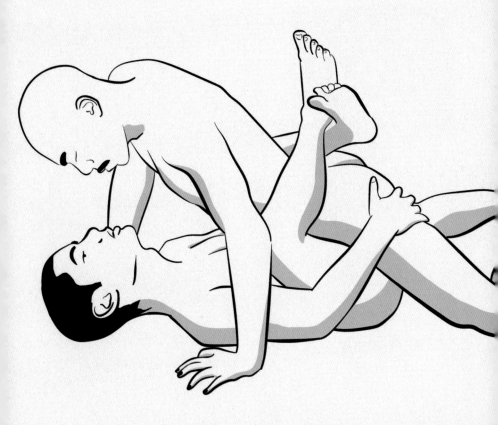

14

The Union like a Crab

An intense version of missionary.

How to Do It

The receiver lies on their back, crossing their legs and lifting them up to their stomach. The giver kneels by their partner's butt with their knees spread widely apart. The giver can either keep their legs tucked under them or bend them behind them along the bed. The receiver wraps their legs around their partner's waist, crossing their ankles behind their partner's back. (Like . . . a crab? Maybe?) The giver keeps their back straight and bends slightly over their partner's body, holding them by their knees, or lying further over their body and resting their weight on their hands.

What's Good About It

This has all the good stuff about missionary—it's face to face, and everyone pretty much knows what to do—but the receiver can wrap their legs around their partner and pull them tighter, which is the international sign for "I want you even deeper."

Tweak It

The giver can mix penetration with breakout sessions to give the receiver oral sex.

Make It Even Better

Start off by giving each other a leisurely massage beforehand. Fire up some candles and use a luxe scented oil (keep oils out of vaginas). Make it more relaxing and spa-like with a massage candle that melts into massage oil or preheat the massage oil in a bowl of warm water.

15

The Churning of the Cream

Whip it, whip it good.

How to Do It

Okay. *cracks knuckles* Let's do this. The receiver lies on their back and rolls back onto their shoulders, pulling their legs as far over their head as they can and spreading their arms on either side for balance. The giver squats above their partner, feet on either side. The giver has their hands pressing down on their partner's thighs, both for balance and for deep penetration. The giver looks like they're sitting on their partner's butt, but it's more of a hover where they hold their weight up with their feet and thigh muscles.

What's Good About It

If you're willing to do the hard positioning stuff, this feels very intense and X-rated whether you do it anally or vaginally. Plus the receiver gets a bit of a head rush.

Tweak It

If the receiver hasn't been doing their shoulder stands in yoga, they can use a wall or the side of a couch or bed for stability.

Make It Even Better

Vary the thrusts. The receiver can rock their hips up a little or swivel them. The giver can make that cream with the up-and-down churning motion or small circles with their hips.

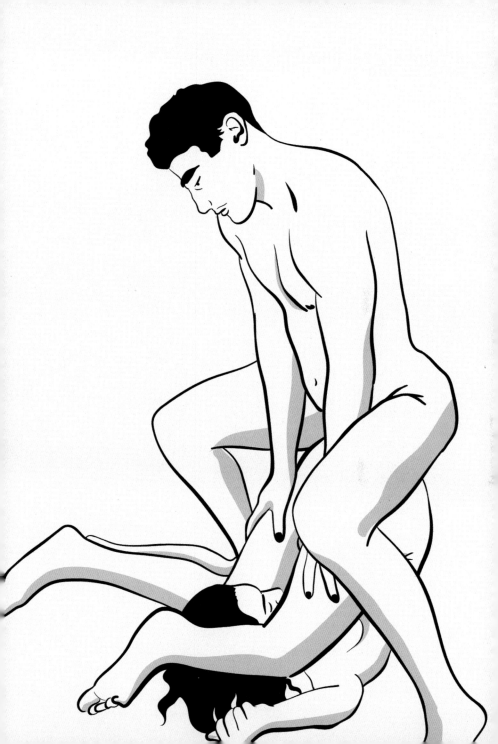

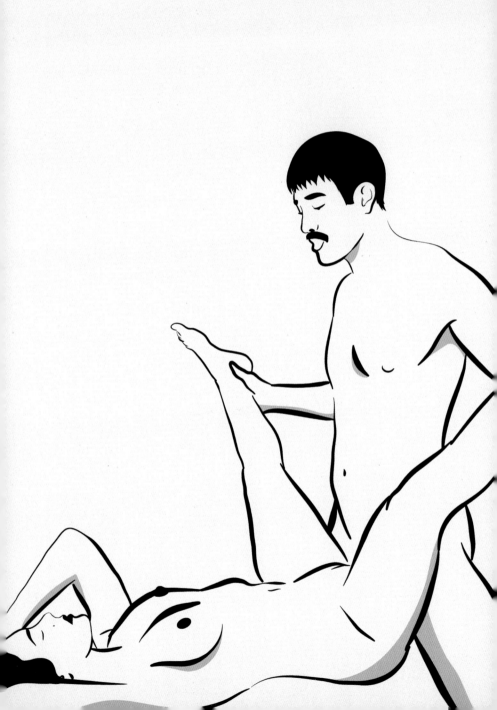

16 The Flag of Cupid

Open up and say aaaaahhh.

How to Do It

The receiver lies on their back with their legs straight up in the air in a V shape. The giver kneels between the partner's legs and takes an ankle in each hand, spreading their thighs apart and holding their legs. For better leverage and more comfort, the giver can also stand next to the bed.

What's Good About It

Whether you're going in anally or vaginally, the Flag of Cupid offers extremely deep penetration, lots of internal stimulation for the receiver, and a really great view for both people.

Tweak It

The giver can move the receiver's legs to change the angles—press the legs together, hold both to one side, or open and shut them like scissors to experiment with what feels best.

Make It Even Better

Indulge your tendencies toward voyeurism and/or exhibitionism. The receiver can teasingly play with themselves with their hands or a toy, pinch their nipples, or just close their eyes, throw their head back, and bring themselves to a thundering orgasm. It can be a huge turn-on to know you are being watched or to watch your partner in the throes of orgasm while you are inside of them.

17

The Flower in Bloom

Spread 'em.

How to Do It

The receiver lies on their back, puts their hands under their butt, and lifts their hips, like the bridge pose in yoga. The receiver spreads their thighs as wide apart as they can while keeping their feet as close to their hips as they can. The giver kneels or crouches by their partner's butt, or, if they're feeling lazy, they can sit with their legs straight out.

What's Good About It

Deep penetration, G- or P-spot stimulation, and either person can use a hand or toy to stimulate the receiver's junk.

Tweak It

Try some nipple play. The receiver can play with their own nipples, or the giver can squeeze and stroke their partner's nipples. Or take it more hardcore with some nipple clamps.

Make It Even Better

If you want to make this more BDSM, the giver can keep the receiver in position with a sex wedge to keep their hips propped up and a spreader bar (a bar that keeps a person's knees apart) between their legs. Not only does the receiver get to completely submit to their partner, which is its own kind of fun, the wedge keeps their hips elevated so they don't have to work very hard to maintain the bridge position.

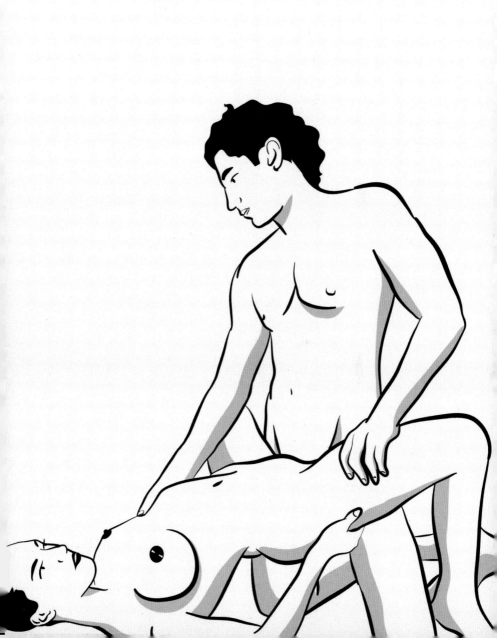

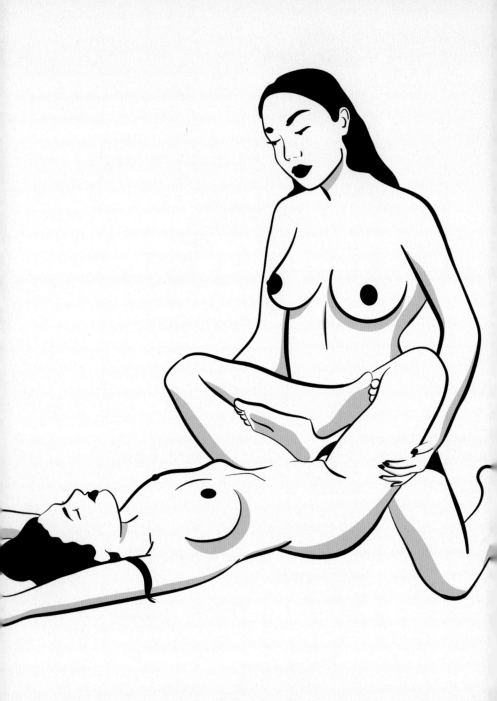

18 Indrani

The Kama Sutra is all about making it twisty.

How to Do It

The receiver lies on their back with their legs crossed or, if they're feeling it, the full-on lotus position (legs crossed with each foot on the opposite thigh). If that's not happening, the receiver can draw their legs up as far as they'll go so their calves touch their thighs and their knees touch their chest. If THAT'S not happening (reasonable!), the receiver just lifts their legs however they damn well please. The giver kneels so they're penetrating while pressing against their partner's thighs to open their legs wide.

What's Good About It

Since the giver is pressing their partner's legs open, it tilts the receiver's pelvis up so it's resting against the giver's legs and opens up their hips. If the receiver has a vulva, this gives their clit more contact with their partner's pelvic bone.

Tweak It

For deeper penetration, or if the receiver's legs are tired, they can unfold their legs and put them up onto their partner's chest.

Make It Even Better

A couple's vibrator will zhuzh this position up for both of you. Try something wearable for hands-free buzzy love.

19

The Lotus-Like Position

Lotus-ish for the less flexible.

How to Do It

The receiver lies on their back with their feet on their thighs in the lotus position (legs crossed with each foot on the opposite side) or with legs crossed in whatever way feels comfortable. The giver leans over their partner's body, holding themselves on knees and hands.

What's Good About It

This position makes it easy to gaze lovingly at each other while you get your sex on. Looking into each other's eyes while you move together makes everything 89.3 percent hotter.

Tweak It

Lean into the romance. The receiver can love up their partner by stroking their face and shoulders and playing with their nipples.

Make It Even Better

This is a good anal position, especially for beginners, because the receiver can control how deep the penis or strap-on goes. The receiver can slow it down or back it up a bit by pressing their feet and calves against their partner's belly. As with all anal, make sure the receiver is well aroused and very ready before doing any penetration; go very slowly, letting the receiver guide the speed; and use a ton of lube (look for a version designed for anal sex) since butts aren't self-lubricating.

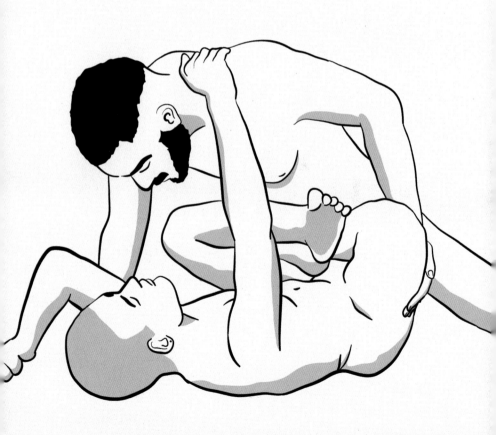

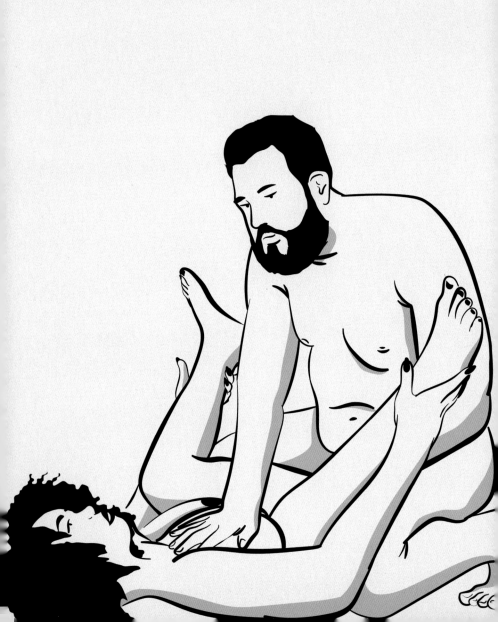

20

The Monkey

I want to F you like an animal.

How to Do It

The receiver rocks onto their back, holding onto their ankles in each of their hands as they raise their feet. (The receiver is supposed to do this "with a mischievous grin," but you do you.) The giver crouches monkey-like between their partner's legs. The giver can slap and kiss their partner's chest playfully before penetrating, but OPTIONAL with the slapping bit.

What's Good About It

The Kama Sutra is big on animal inspiration for positions to harness the essence of various animals. This one is all about playfulness, laughing, and having fun. Sex is silly—there are accidental elbows in the face, random queefs and farts, and general awkwardness. Embrace that and have a good laugh together.

Tweak It

Both of you can make whatever primitive animal sounds you're feeling. Maybe hot? Maybe just silly? Find out.

Make It Even Better

Get in touch with your monkey selves by taking turns wielding a vibrator and acting like you don't know what it's for. Press it against each other's chests, hands, thighs, and inner arms and see what happens. People with vulvas usually like vibrators on or near their clits or against their vulvas. People with penises might like a vibrator pressed against the bottom of the shaft or their perineum (the area between the balls and the butt hole.) Be curious like George.

THE POSITIONS

21

The Union of Fixing a Nail

Bang, bang.

How to Do It

The receiver lies on their back with one leg outstretched along the bed. They raise their other leg, putting their foot on their partner's forehead. The giver kneels between their partner's thighs, pressing against their thigh as they thrust.

What's Good About It

The giver is in a great position to squeeze the receiver's thigh, stroke their chest or rub their penis or vulva with a hand or a toy. If the receiver would rather rub themselves, that works too. The receiver can also massage their partner's thighs or squeeze their ass affectionately.

Tweak It

To switch up sensations, the giver can raise or lower the angle of penetration by scooting up or down, and the receiver can switch it up and control the depth by pressing their foot more lightly or harder against their partner's forehead.

Make It Even Better

This is an excellent position for foot play. The giver can kiss the soles of their partner's feet, lick the arch, or take each toe in their mouth and suck on it. If one among you happens to have a foot fetish (or are looking to develop one) this position is *insert fire emoji*.

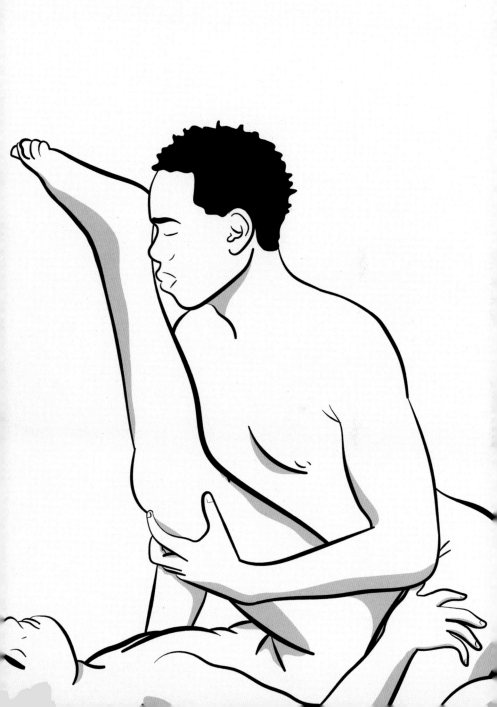

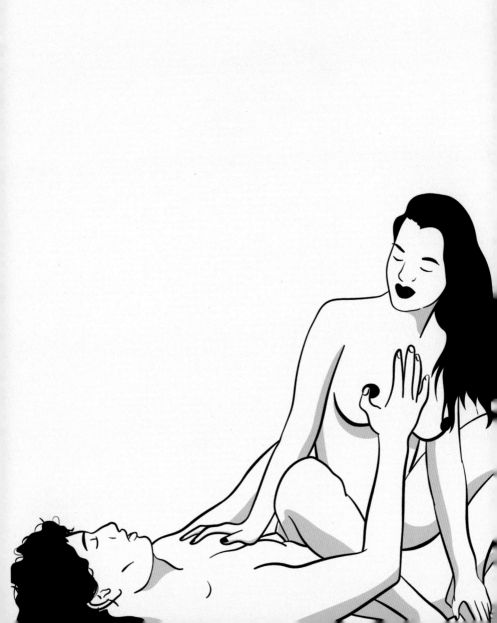

22

The Union of the Spinning Top

You spin me round like a record.

How to Do It

The giver lies flat on the bed, legs slightly spread. The receiver squats over their partner, facing them and straddling their torso. The receiver keeps their feet at their partner's sides with knees up and their partner's penis or strap-on inside their vagina or anus and begins to ride. This, my friend, is just the beginning. *Then* the receiver turns carefully to one side, keeping their partner inside them while they turn. Once situated, the receiver rides as they please. The receiver repeats the turns until they've done a full 360.

What's Good About It

This is just a fun way to experiment with different feelz. Plus, the person on top gets to control the motion so they can move however they want to and be the boss of everything.

Tweak It

This requires some coordination to keep the contact going. The giver can give a literal hand by helping lift their partner to the next spot.

Make It Even Better

The receiver can experiment with a different motion at each "stop" on the route. Try leaning backward or forward, rocking, squeezing, and/or riding up and down.

THE POSITIONS

23

The Union like a Swing

Even the ancients knew of the powers of reverse cowgirl.

How to Do It

The giver lies on their back, resting on their arms or using pillows behind the arms and back for support. The receiver straddles their partner's hips facing away from them and rests their hands on their partner's calves or thighs.

What's Good About It

The Kama Sutra's version of cowgirl has the receiver doing a gentle rocking or swinging motion instead of the usual up or down thrusting. No eye contact, but the giver gets a nice ass-side view.

Tweak It

To mix it up or if the person on top's thighs are giving out, the receiver can rise up on all fours so they're hovering instead of sitting on their partner. The receiver rubs themselves with a hand or toy while the giver thrusts up into them for internal and external stimulation.

Make It Even Better

If the receiver wants to be the World's Best Lover, they can contract their Kegel muscles or their anus around their partner's penis, squeezing and holding in sync with their rocking. (If their partner has a strap-on, this move is way less World's Best but will still enhance it for the receiver.)

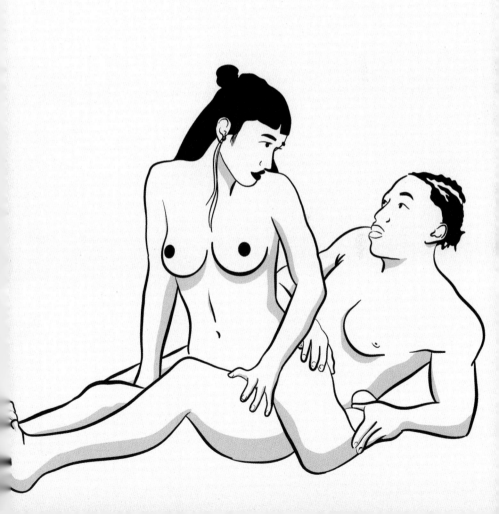

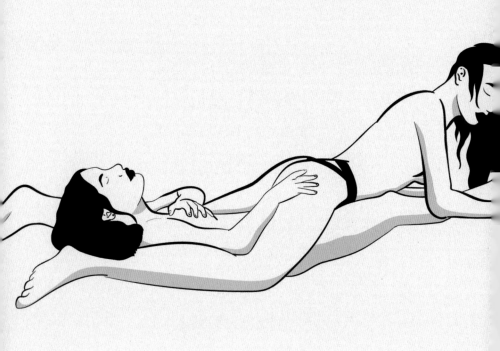

24 The Turning Union with Giver on Top

Dramamine optional.

How to Do It

The receiver lies on their back with their legs stretched out in front of them and slightly spread. The giver lies on top of their partner and enters missionary style, pumping away as long as they'd like. BUT like The Union of the Spinning Top (page 59), there's MORE. Slowly and carefully, the giver turns themselves around—keeping their penis or strap-on inside their partner—so their head is between their partner's feet and their feet are one either side of their partner's head. Try that for a bit, then return, doing 180s as long as y'all want.

What's Good About It

This is kind of a novelty position but is great for exploring what feels good to you both. If it's some upside 180 position like this, then—huzzah!—you've learned a new thing.

Tweak It

If you have two vulvas onboard, a flexible double-headed dildo is great for handling the turns.

Make It Even Better

This can be not especially comfortable or actually painful if the receiver has a vulva. Try a version without the 180, where the giver is lying perpendicularly to the receiver instead. Still fun, less hurty. (If anything feels off during sex, either of you should feel free to stop, any time, no questions asked.)

25 The Full-Pressed Union

Push it real good.

How to Do It

The receiver lies on their back and the giver kneels in front. The receiver pulls their legs up so they're resting on their partner's thighs, then bends their knees, pulling their thighs to their chest. The receiver then presses the soles of their feet against their partner's chest.

What's Good About It

This positions you both for deep penetration, either anally or vaginally. The receiver can easily change the depth and intensity by how hard they press their feet against their partner's chest.

Tweak It

The giver can use their hands to rub their partner's thighs, feet, and calves, or if they want to get in *really* good, ply their partner's penis or vulva with a hand or toy. For a tighter feel, the receiver can press their legs together.

Make It Even Better

Indulge in some dom/sub play (with enthusiastic consent, always) by having the giver control the motion by holding their partner's hips and rocking them back and forth, using their partner's body like a sex toy or Fleshlight. The dom can assert their control verbally with commands such as "Squeeze that little ass/pussy for me" or making the sub beg for more.

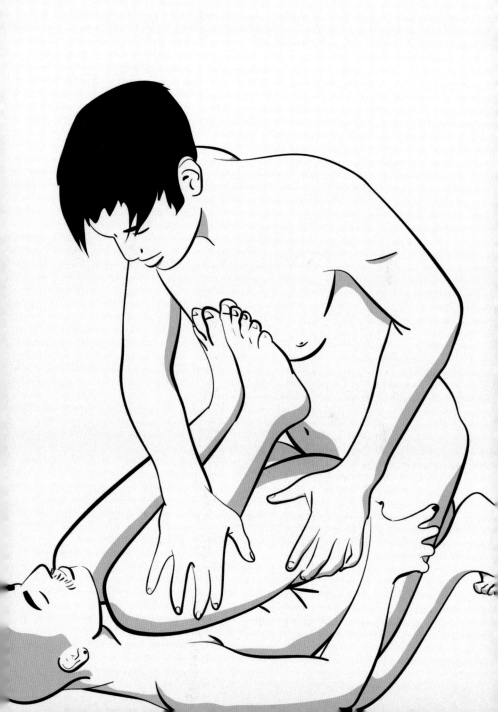

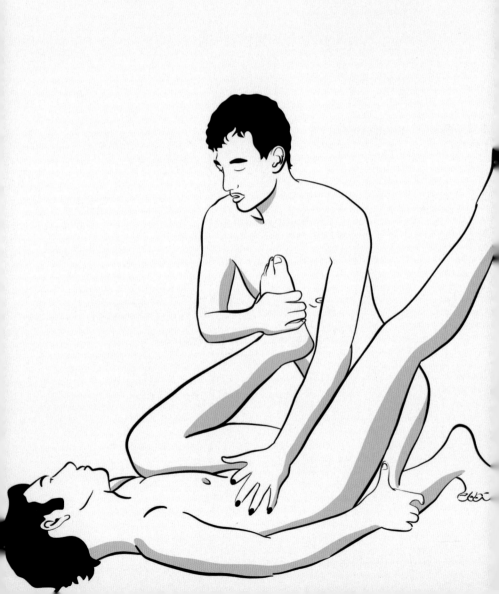

26 The Half-Pressed Union

Get a leg up.

How to Do It

The receiver lies on their back and the giver kneels by their hips. The giver raises their partner's hips onto their thighs, and the receiver pulls their thighs to their chest until penetration. Then the receiver puts one foot on their partner's chest and stretches the other legs straight out, over their partner's thighs. As the giver thrusts, the receiver moves their straight leg up and down.

What's Good About It

This position gives both partners a chance to control the motion. The giver has plenty of leeway to do whatever kind of thrusting they're feeling, and the receiver can adjust the angle and feel of the penetration by lifting their straight leg up and down and twisting their hips a bit.

Tweak It

The receiver can play with switching back and forth between which leg is the straight one to mix up the sensations.

Make It Even Better

Throw down some old towels or blankets and douse yourselves in copious amounts of lube. Smear it on each other's chests, cover your thighs and bellies, and slather lube between each other's legs. Run your hands and bodies all over each other's slipperiness. Afterward you can hit the shower together.

27 The Packed Union

Pay a visit to the meat packing factory.

How to Do It

The receiver lies on their back, crossing their legs at the ankles. They pull their legs up and keep their thighs together and close to their chest so they can rest their feet on their partner's chest. The giver kneels at their partner's hips to enter and holds on tight.

What's Good About It

The whole series of the Kama Sutra "union" poses are great for deep penetration, either anally or vaginally, and allow one or both partners to have a hand free to stimulate themselves or the other person. They also give the receiver a raised foot or two to use so they can guide how deep they want to take a penis or strap-on.

Tweak It

Try it with a vibrating cock ring. The ring traps blood in the penis, keeping it harder, and will provide rumbly vibes to both partners. If a strap-on is involved, hardness is not a factor, but the vibes still feel good.

Make It Even Better

Try a dom/sub scenario with the person on the bottom calling the shots. They can issue commands such as "Faster," "Nice and slow," "Suck my toes," or whatever they want their obedient little sub to do.

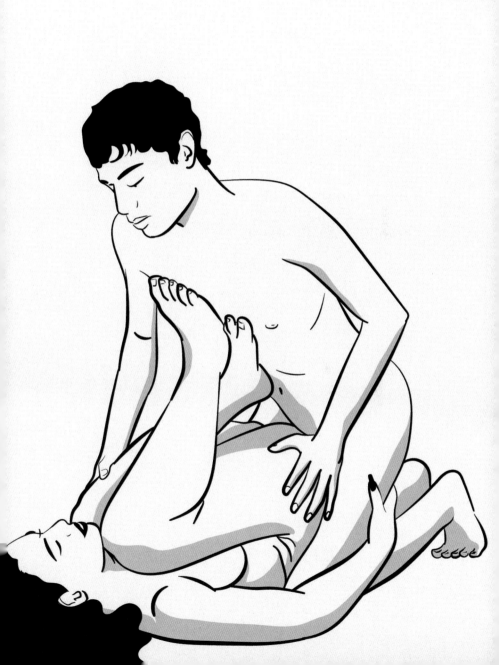

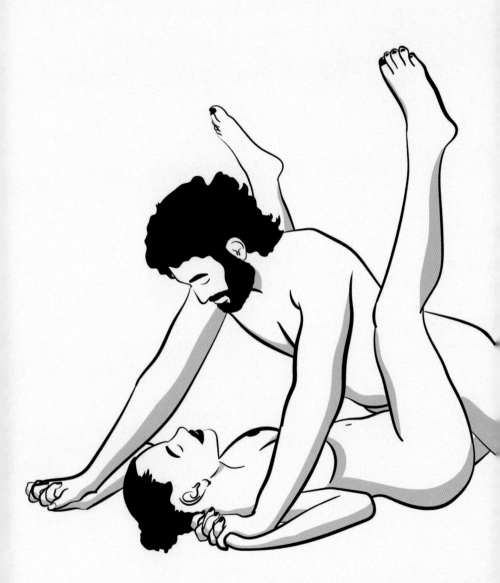

28

The Yawning Position

As in open wide, not ZZZZZ.

How to Do It

The receiver lies on their back with their legs straight up in the air. The giver gets on their hands and knees and leans over their partner's body. The two partners press the palms of their hands together and look into each other's eyes.

What's Good About It

The easy access deep penetration is great, but making the point to press your hands together and gaze into each other's eyes helps you lock in and makes this position feel more intimate and connected.

Tweak It

Want to go even deeper??? Is this even scientifically possible? Yes! If the receiver has the flexibility, they can put their legs up over their partner's shoulders, and (carefully) explore those depths.

Make It Even Better

The Kama Sutra is big on teaching vulva-pleasing. Warm up a yoni by playing with the hood of the clit. Gently push and pull it, twist it between your wet fingers, or tap it. Slowly unveil the clit, then tease it by flicking, tapping, or holding it between two fingers. Work up to a firmer rub. Then try going in circles or rubbing your hand back and forth across the clit or over the whole vulva.

29 The Yawning Position—Variation

Like the regular old Yawning Position, but even DEEPER.

How to Do It

The receiver lies on their back, holding their legs in the air with their feet on each side of their partner's head. The giver gets on their hands and knees and leans over their partner's body to enter.

What's Good About It

Lots! Face-to-face contact, insanely deep penetration, much eye gazing, and a choice of two holes to ravish. (PSA: Never put anything in a vagina after it's been in a butt. Vagina to butt, however, is A-OK.)

Tweak It

Give it a BDSM-adjacent vibe by having the giver press their partner's hand to the bed, pinning them down.

Make It Even Better

Like the regular Yawning Position, and all positions for that matter, it's gonna go better if everyone is well aroused before any penetration happens. For a vulva, try sliding a wet flat palm over the vulva, bringing the palm slowly upward then back down. Slide a curled finger inside the vagina and press it against the upper wall. For a penis, stroke the shaft with a wet hand, making a twisting motion as you go up and down, being sure to make a pass over the head on the down stroke.

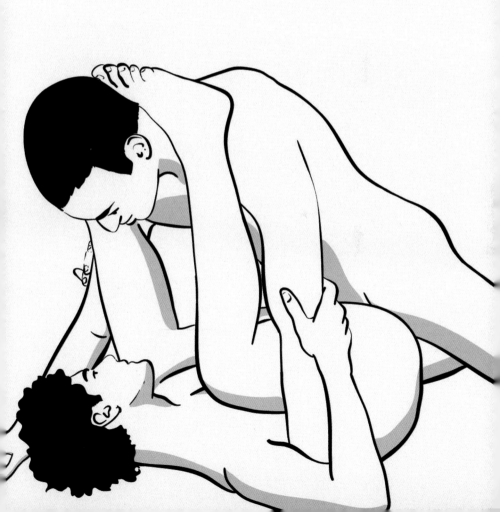

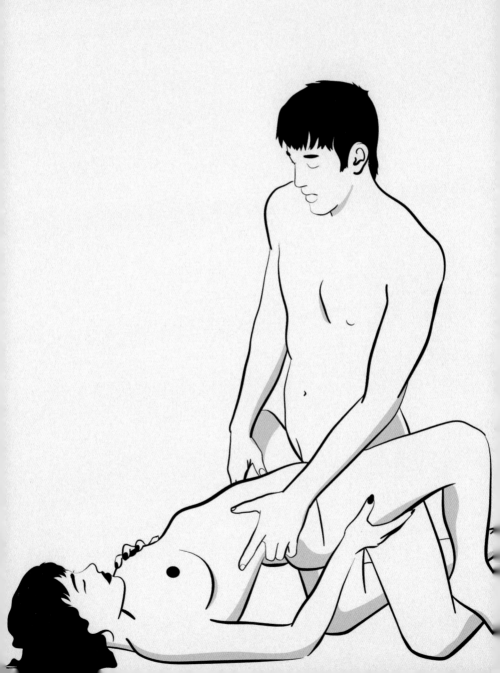

30

The Widely Opened Position

Think reverse hip-dips.

How to Do It

The receiver lies on their back with their feet on the bed, then pushes their hips into the air. They keep their knees bent and their shoulders and upper arms on the bed. The giver kneels between their legs to enter. The receiver can keep their feet on the bed or lift them up so they're resting on their partner's thighs.

What's Good About It

This allows both people to thrust and grind gainst each other, plus the giver has their hands free and can easily stroke their partner wherever they might need stroking.

Tweak It

If it's hard for the receiver to maintain the position, they've got options. The giver can hold their hips up with their hands. The receiver can support themselves on their hands and arms by holding their butt. Or you can bust out some positioning pillows and let them handle it.

Make It Even Better

Make a game of it by challenging each other with your thrusts. Try something—shallow and quick, slow circles, deep and hard—and see if your partner can match it. Or take turns doing the moving while your partner stays still and enjoys the ride.

31 The Wife of Indra

Thank you, o nameless wife of yore.

How to Do It

The receiver lies on their back with their knees tucked up to their chest. They hold their knees with their hands, keeping them close to the chest and spread slightly. The giver kneels between their partner's legs and leans over, putting their hands by their partner's shoulders. The receiver can put their feet at their partner's sides or on their belly.

What's Good About It

This a good position for givers with smaller penises or strap-ons because they can get on in there. Givers who are packing large should be careful and check with their partner to make sure it's not painful.

Tweak It

Make it a little weird by having the receiver put their feet into their partner's armpits for leverage.

Make It Even Better

Channel the spirit of Indra's wife. Indra was a Vedic king whose wife was known for creating new and interesting ways to have sex, and this was supposedly his favorite. (Not sure how they all knew this—pre-TMZ, no less.) Figure out something you can do to make this position your favorite. Is it anal with a G-spot toy? Telling each other a dirty, dirty fantasy as you move? Up to you!

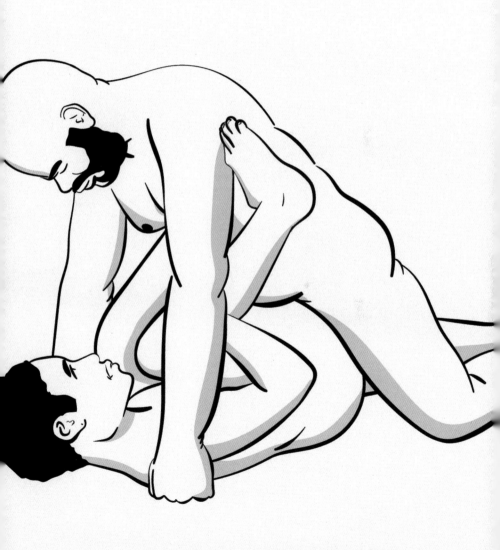

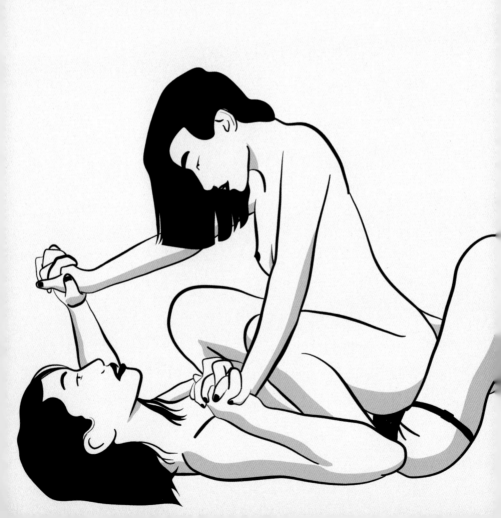

32

The Amazon

Like cowgirl, but more squatty.

How to Do It

The giver lies on their back with their knees bent. The receiver squats over their partner, putting their feet on either side of their hips. The giver wraps their feet around their partner's hips or, if their body doesn't go that way, just keeps their legs splayed out in whatever way feels comfortable. Hold hands for support and/or bonding.

What's Good About It

This one lets the receiver take complete control of the motion, the speed, the depth—everything. Whatever they want, they get. The receiver can be a kindly overlord and stroke their partner's chest and play with their nipples as they move.

Tweak It

The receiver can muck about with their strokes. They can sway or circle their hips or move up and down to thrust (careful, though: Penis breakage is a real thing that can happen).

Make It Even Better

If you want to try some role-play, the Amazon is a good place to start. Professor and student? Doctor and patient? A pizza delivery person scenario? Role-play can be whatever you want. It doesn't have to be anything moral or acceptable IRL. In fact, it might even be better if it's not. Go ahead and play with the forbidden.

33 The Feet Yoke

Mirror, mirror.

How to Do It

The receiver sits straight on the bed, folding one leg under themselves so they're sitting on it and extending the other leg along the bed. The giver mirrors their partner, putting their folded leg over the partner's extended leg and under their folded leg. Wrap your arms around each other for balance or put a hand on the bed.

What's Good About It

This position is hard to get into, which can be its own kind of fun. It's bonding to work together to do something hard. Plus, the closeness of your bodies and the eye contact makes it feel even more connected.

Tweak It

This isn't great for hard and fast thrusting so embrace the slow and shallow penetration. Rock and grind against each other, sliding a hand or two down to help out if you'd like.

Make It Even Better

If this isn't gonna be enough orgasmic stimulation for one of both of you, switch to mutual masturbation. For a vulva, try inserting two or three fingers inside the vagina, using the thumb to rub across or around the clit. Alternate pressure and deep thrusting or vibrating your hand. For a penis, try the 7-and-1 stroke. Stroke upward along the shaft for seven strokes, then a single downward stroke, and repeat.

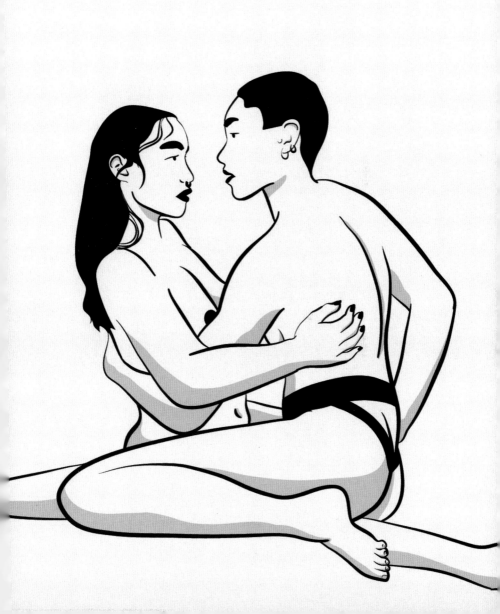

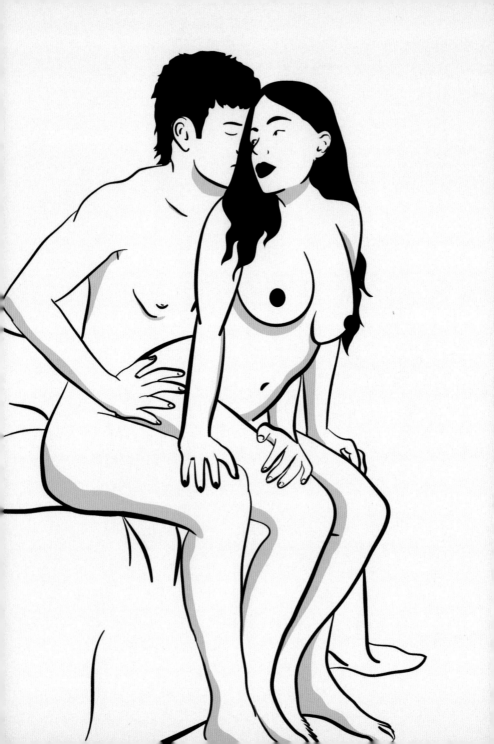

34 The Knot of Fame

Have a seat.

How to Do It

The giver sits upright on the edge of a sofa, chair, or bed. The receiver sits on their partner's lap facing away from them to ride. The receiver has their feet on the floor and hands on the chair arms or mattress for leverage.

What's Good About It

This is fun variation for penetrative sex anally or vaginally, but it's also convenient for a reach around. And if the receiver is shy, has sensory issues, or just doesn't like eye contact, they're all set.

Tweak It

For a nonpenetrative option, have the giver lavish their full attention on their lap-sitter. They can play with their partner's nipples and squeeze or spank their ass while stroking their penis or vulva. Add neck and ear kisses and some whispered filthiness or words of love. Afterward the receiver can return the favor.

Make It Even Better

The Kama Sutra says that the loins and thighs should slap together, like the sound of an "elephant's ears." Go hard with the animalistic aspect and slap those body parts together, make some noise, moan loudly, and let go of your inhibitions.

35

The Lotus

Bend and then bend some more.

How to Do It

Both partners sit face-to-face. The giver sits with their legs bent and the bottoms of their feet pressed together. The receiver wraps their legs around the giver's neck—the giver can provide a little help here—then crosses their ankles and holds onto their toes.

What's Good About It

Because of the angle of your bodies, this is an excellent anal position. But regardless of how y'all go in, this is an intimate position that requires trust, flexibility and, if it doesn't quite work out, a sense of humor.

Tweak It

Since there's not a lot of motion in this one, amp up the stimulation with an arousal oil or warming or cooling lube.

Make It Even Better

Adjust, adjust, adjust. This is a hard position to get into and a hard one to maintain. You don't get any points for doing it "right," so do whatever you need to do to make it work for you. The giver doesn't *have* to press their feet together—put 'em another way if it feels better. If the receiver's legs only want to go up to the giver's chest instead of their neck—congratulations!—you've discovered your own new position.

KAMA SUTRA NIGHTS

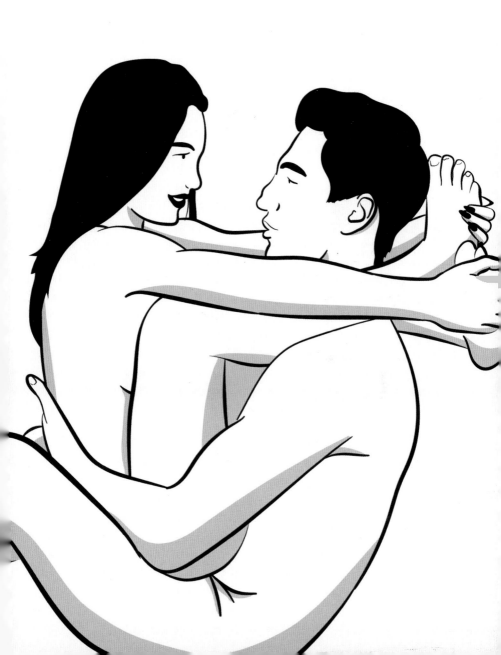

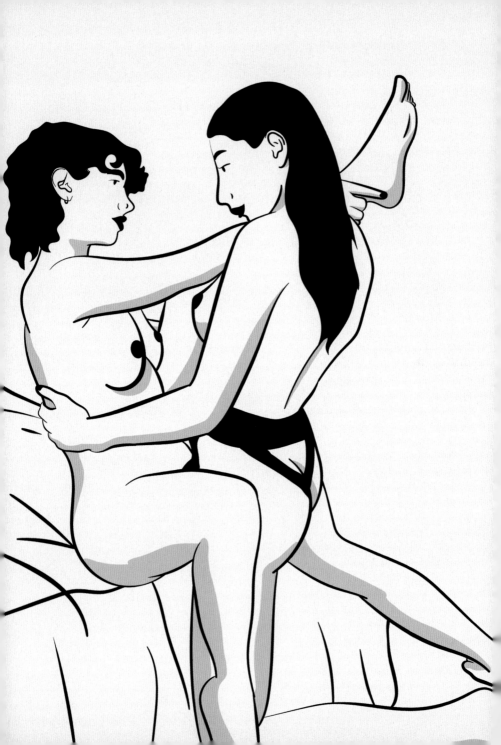

36

The Peacock

The splits plus sex.

How to Do It

The receiver perches on the edge of a bed or chair and raises one leg up as straight as possible, holding onto their ankle with their hands. The other foot is on the floor. The giver kneels or squats on the floor to enter. The giver is in charge of providing the balance.

What's Good About It

If the giver is into legs, hey, they have a whole leg right there to enjoy. Plus the receiver is slightly off-balance, which adds a little shot of adrenaline.

Tweak It

The giver can lavish the receiver's raised leg with the attention it deserves. Try kisses on the ankle, licks behind the knee, and nibbles up the inner thigh.

Make It Even Better

Prioritize comfort. If the receiver doesn't want to make their leg go straight, they can bend it or wrap it around their partner's waist. Plop a pillow or two for the giver to kneel on to protect their knees. If a chair isn't the right height, try a bed instead. Or do a version with the receiver on the table and the giver standing. Find something that works for you both.

37 The Swing

Maybe not the kind of swinging you're thinking of.

How to Do It

Both partners sit down and face each other. The giver has their legs out in front of them, knees bent. The giver sits on the receiver's lap facing their partner and wraps their legs around their partner's hips. Hold onto each other's wrists or hands and lean back. Take turns leaning back, pulling the other person forward, rocking back and forth like you're on a seesaw. The movement is gentle and smooth.

What's Good About It

This position relies on deep connection and trust—it's not the kind of thing you'd bust out during a hookup. It focuses your attention on each other so you get the incredibly intimate experience of watching someone go toward, then through, an orgasm.

Tweak It

This is great as a nonpenetrative position. You can scooch a little toward or away from each other to adjust it. Try it with each of you touching yourselves (either simultaneously or take turns) or reach for each other for mutual handies.

Make It Even Better

Make it an ultra-bonding experience by agreeing not to talk during it. Just stare into each other's eyes and feel your bodies rocking together. (Moaning and sighing are completely allowed.)

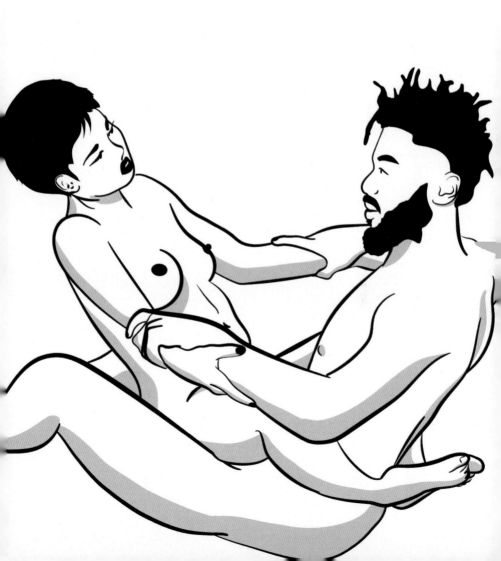

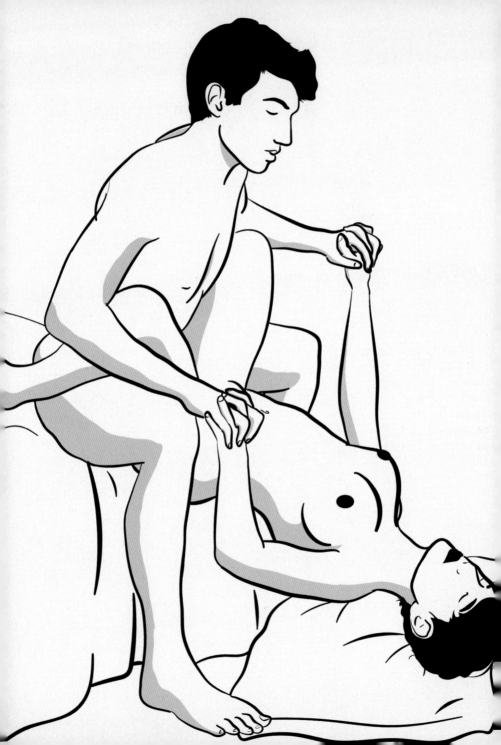

38

The Trapeze

Step right up for this amazing feat!

How to Do It

The giver sits at the edge of a bed or chair. The receiver sits on their partner's lap and straddles them, sliding onto their penis or strap-on. Holding hands, the receiver slowly leans back until they are hanging upside down (cue circus music). For balance, the receiver can hook their legs around their partner's waist or hips.

What's Good About It

The thrill of doing a head rush-inducing acrobatic feat, plus you get to bond over the shared experience of making this tricky position work.

Tweak It

Be safe. The giver needs to hold on firmly and confidently to help the receiver be able to relinquish control and lean back. No one's gonna be dropping anyone, but . . . scattering a few pillows on the ground will help the receiver feel more confident about relaxing into the position.

Make It Even Better

If a vulva is involved, this position will require some extra clit stimulation. Since no one's hands will be free—they're making sure the brave trapeze artist does not plunge to the floor—try a wearable panty vibe or a couple's vibrator that provides internal G-spot stimulation coupled with an external part that fits against the clit.

39

The Union like a Pair of Tongs

But like, sexy tongs.

How to Do It

The giver lies on their back, legs comfortably extended in front of them. The receiver straddles their partner with one leg on either side and feet tucked under their partner's butt. The receiver rocks gently against their partner's body.

What's Good About It

This is a slow, sexy position where most of the movement is going on internally. The "tongs" in the title refer to yoni squeezing a lingam—but this can work with the receiver squeezing their Kegel muscles or tightening their anus. (Mini Kegel refresher: To find your Kegel muscles, tighten your pelvic muscles like you're trying not to pee. Feel that? Congratulations—you have discovered your Kegel muscles!)

Tweak It

Sync the squeezes to the rocking motions or try varying them, shifting between long squeezes and quick fluttering. The receiver can close those tongs even more by squeezing their thighs together.

Make It Even Better

Both of you have a great chance to use your hands on each other. The receiver can rub their partner's shoulders and arms, stroke their chest, or lean over and lick and kiss their nipples. The giver can reach up and stroke their partner's chest or squeeze their thighs or stroke their penis or vulva.

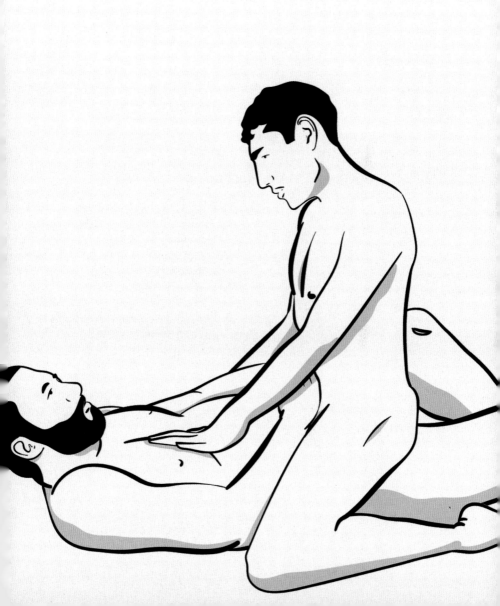

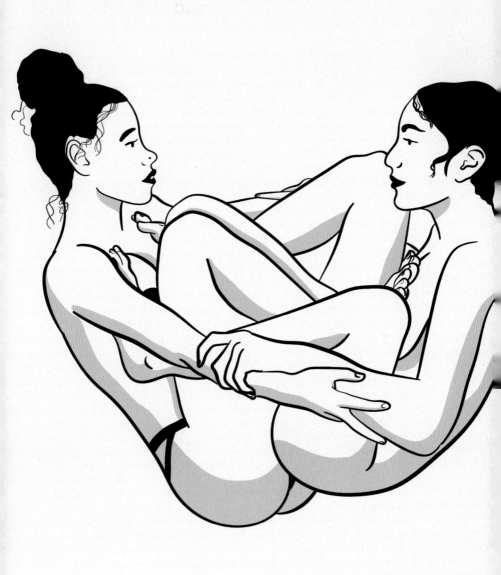

40

The Tortoise

Slow and steady wins the race.

How to Do It

Both partners sit face-to-face and lift their feet to play with each other's nipples. Then they take hold of each other's forearms or hands and scoot forward so that they're butt to butt. The receiver puts their knees together and puts their feet on their partner's chest. The giver puts their legs outside their partner's and puts their feet on their partner's shoulders or chest. Hold hands and look into each other's eyes.

What's Good About It

This position is about mirroring, so it enhances intimacy. It's designed for penetration, and you can certainly try for that, but this position is very advanced.

Tweak It

If it's not working, try a plan B. Have the giver sit cross-legged, or for extra yogi bonus points, in the lotus position. The receiver sits on their partner's lap and presses their chests together. Then put your heads together and touch lips.

Make It Even Better

You can go hard on the spirituality and mirroring aspect of this with lots of eye gazing and visualizing energy flowing between you. Or you can use it as kind of a boob footsie foreplay, then slide over on top of your partner for something more genitally focused.

41

The Peddling Tortoise

Deep breaths, everyone.

How to Do It

Both people sit face-to-face. The receiver raises one hand in the air and wraps the leg on the same side around their partner's waist. The giver mirrors their partner, hand on their partner's hand and leg around their partner's waist. Feel free to stop there. Truly, it's okay—our illustrated couple did! However, for bonus points, both people then lift the other foot and press those together in front of them as well, moving their feet together like they're peddling.

What's Good About It

The fun of this is in the trying. If you can actually do it, good on you. You'll probably have better luck if you skip the foot peddling part, but go ahead and give it a go.

Tweak It

Instead of penetration, use this pose to gaze into each other's eyes and stroke each other.

Make It Even Better

The Kama Sutra describes many different kinds of kisses. This is a good pose to try some of them out. The throbbing kiss is when the lips touch and you "pulse" the bottom lip. The touching kiss is touching your partner's lips with your tongue like a snake then kissing. The bent deep is a locking kiss with your tongues penetrating fully and hands cupping around the back of each other's neck.

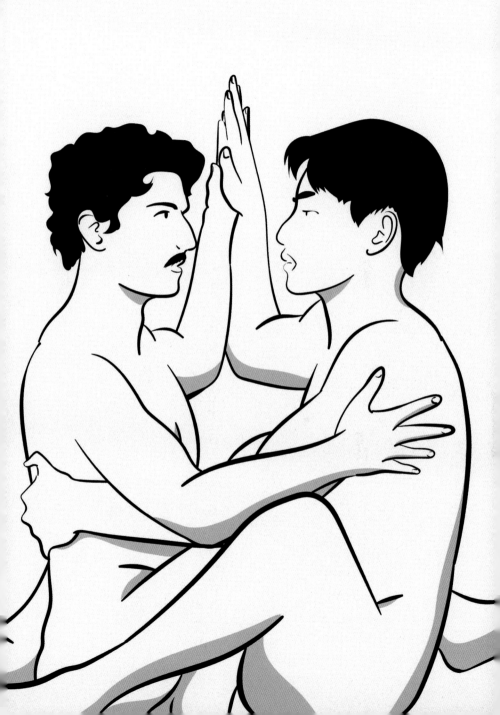

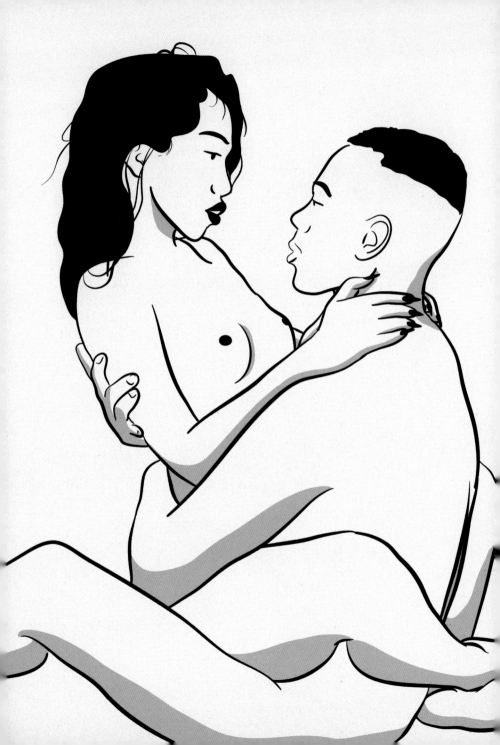

42

The Yab Yum Position

Tantra has entered the chat.

How to Do It

The giver sits with their legs loosely crossed or with legs bent in front of them. The receiver sits on their partner's lap and wraps their legs around their hips. The giver penetrates their partner and the two rock back and forth.

What's Good About It

Yab Yum, which is also a classic Tantric position, is great for fostering deep connection. For people with vulvas, rocking and grinding motion gives more clit stimulation, which can make the position more orgasm-inducing.

Tweak It

Try the Tantric technique of placing your hands on each other's hearts, looking into each other's eyes and synching your breathing. You can touch your foreheads together and feel each other's breath or take the time to indulge in some passionate kissing. When you feel like something spiritual has gone down, you're doing it right.

Make It Even Better

If you're feeling less transcendent and more orgasmy, feel free to reach down to stroke each other, or you can modernize the position with some toys. Depending on what equipment y'all are sporting, you can use vibrating nipple clamps, a strong wand vibrator, vibrating butt plugs for two, a prostate toy, a penis ring, or whatever else does it for you.

43

The Ass

Standing doggie style, STAT.

How to Do It

The receiver stands with their legs apart, with their hands on their thighs for balance. The giver stands behind to enter. For more support, the receiver can stand near a bed, counter, or table and hold the hell on.

What's Good About It

This is an excellent quickie position, the kind of position to use when you don't even want to wait to take your clothes off. Just a quick tug of the pants and it's on.

Tweak It

The receiver can arch their back to change up the angle or press their legs together for a tighter feel. The giver can hold their partner's hips to pull them even closer, reach around and stroke their chest, or knead their ass cheeks.

Make It Even Better

This is great for at-home quickies, but it's even better for forbidden quickies in places where you really shouldn't be having sex. Duck into the restroom of a coffee shop and lean over the sink (make sure there's another restroom available for people who actually need it). Or slip into a spare room, closet, or bathroom at a party and have your way with each other.

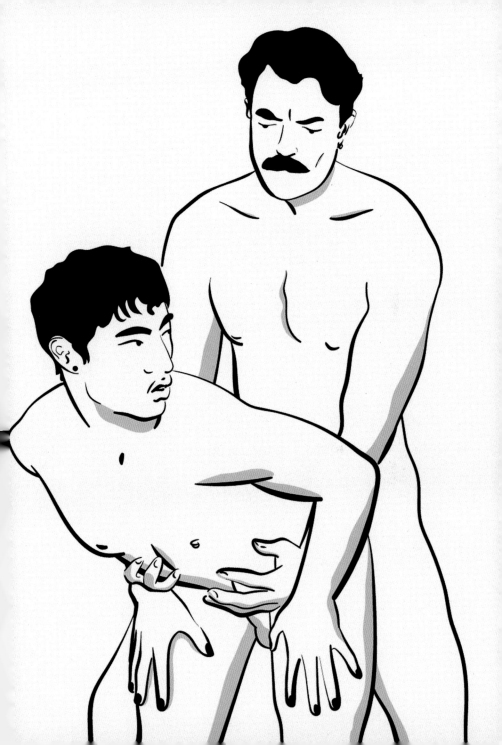

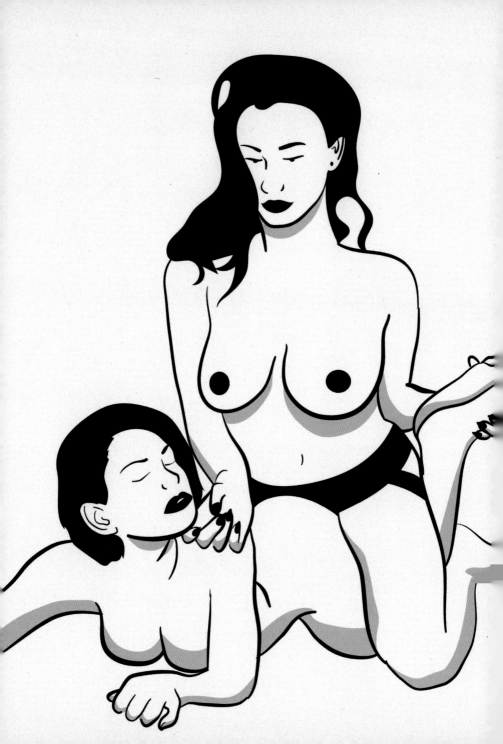

44

The Cat

Meow.

How to Do It

The receiver lies on their stomach, resting their upper torso on their forearms. The giver straddles their partner, holding both of their ankles to the side in one hand. The giver squats or kneels to penetrate and holds onto their partner's chin with the other hand.

What's Good About It

This is twist on typical rear entry positions. The angle is slightly askew, so everything feels a bit different, plus the giver has a bit of dominance over the receiver.

Tweak It

The giver can score extra bonus points by moving both of their hands to the receiver's feet and giving their partner a foot rub while they thrust.

Make It Even Better

In this position, the receiver is supposed to go all-in with the cat concept, rolling around, purring, writhing their hips, and arching their back. If you're both down for it, try a little predator–prey play with the receiver trying to "escape" and the giver trying to capture and pin their prey down. Or see if the giver can pet and stroke this feral kitty to coax them into letting them inside. (Again, big consent all around is necessary with all sex things, but even more so when you're doing something you don't usually do.)

45

The Congress of the Cow

Maybe needs some rebranding, name-wise.

How to Do It

The receiver stands with their legs apart, bending and the waist and putting their hands on the floor. The giver stands behind to penetrate. They can hold onto the receiver's chest, hips, or thighs.

What's Good About It

This is a good position when you want it hard, you want it fast, and you want it now. Also if you happen to be able to touch the floor and want to show off.

Tweak It

Some people want to be pounded while touching their floor, some do not. If the receiver is in that second category, leaning on the back of a couch, table, or bed makes this position waaaay more comfortable/doable.

Make It Even Better

The Kama Sutra stresses the importance of foreplay to raise desire instead of just diving in with the boner-y. For a person with a vulva, the text advises, "The man should rub the yoni of the woman with his hand and fingers (as the elephant rubs anything with his trunk) before engaging in congress, until it is softened, and after that is done he should proceed to put his lingam into her." Heed this wisdom.

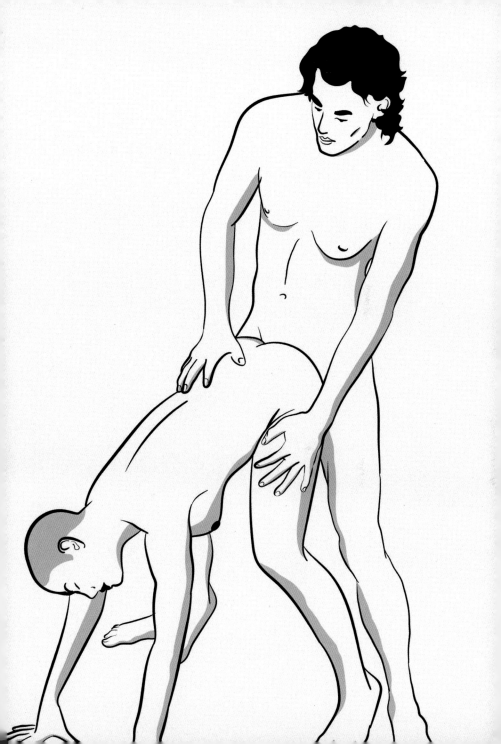

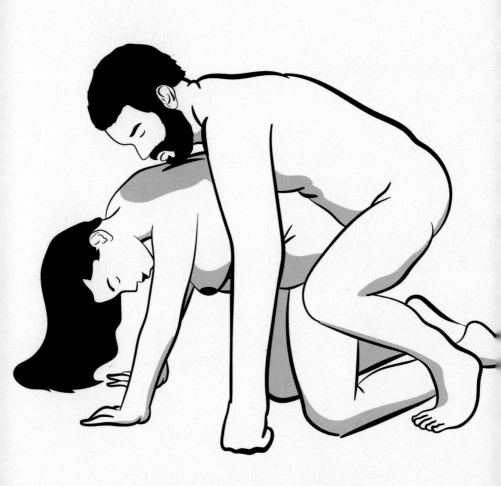

46

The Rutting of the Deer

Like doggie, but more hardcore.

How to Do It

The receiver gets on their hands and knees à la doggie. The giver squats or kneels behind, angling themselves for hard and fast thrusting. The receiver arches their back up and down to create even more movement. Works as a vaginal or anal position.

What's Good About It

Even though the position looks a lot like doggie, it's got a faster, rougher vibe. (Deer apparently like it hard—who knew?) It works best as a finishing move when one or both of you needs to have an orgasm, like, *this very second*.

Tweak It

If the receiver wants more direct stimulation, the giver can do a reach around to service their partner's penis or vulva via hand or toy. A wearable vibrator can also do the job for people with vulvas.

Make It Even Better

Go all-in with the deer rutting theme by making it extra animalistic. Make lots of noise and groan, sigh, and moan filthy/loving things to let each other know how much you're into it. If you've got enthusiastic consent all around (hugely important!), add some playful biting, unnecessary roughness, or a little bit of predator–prey play.

47

The Dog

Or as we call it in modern times, doggie style.

How to Do It

The receiver kneels on their hands and feet with their legs spread slightly. The giver kneels behind, their legs behind their partner's and gripping their waist during penetration.

What's Good About It

Doggie has a primal, animalistic feel that works for quickies, BDSM play, anal sex, or rough, passionate sex.

Tweak It

Doggie is super adjustable, and you can change the mood and/or angles with small changes. For a tighter feel, trade leg positions so that the receiver's legs are inside the giver's and pressed tightly against each other. The receiver can also arch their back up or down to change stimulation for both people. Add an edge of BDSM by having the giver hold onto the receiver's hand to keep them in place or using a spreader bar between the receiver's legs.

Make It Even Better

Doggie is known for being kind of a hardcore position, but you can make it extremely intimate by slowing it way down. The receiver can turn back to gaze at the giver, and the giver can caress the receiver's ass and back. And making it slo-mo helps you both feel *every* inch of each thrust.

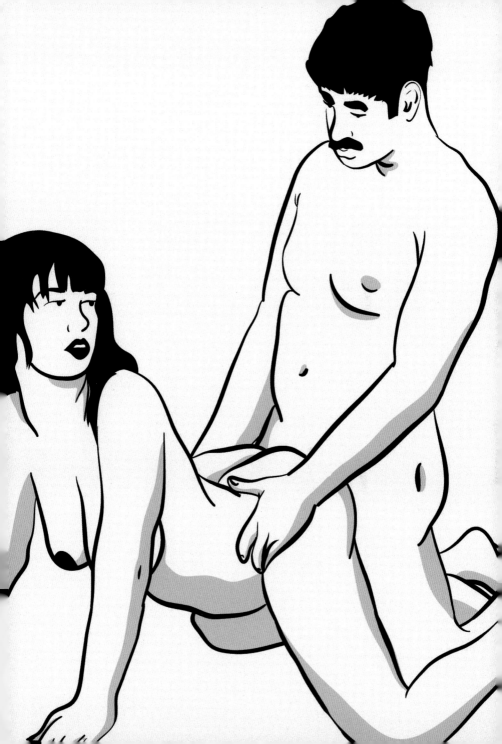

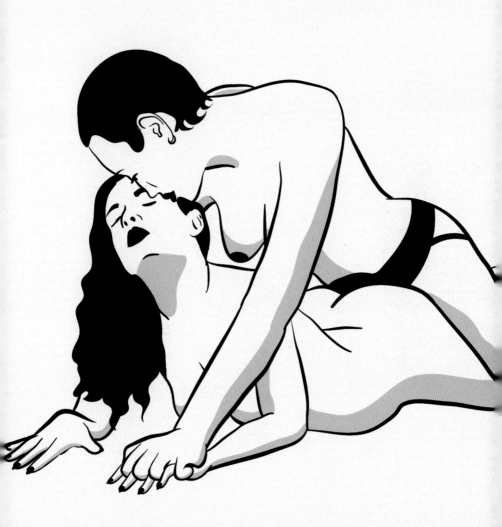

48

The Pressing of the Elephant

Good morning, you.

How to Do It

The receiver lies on their stomach with their legs slightly apart and pelvis lifted. They can support themselves on their forearms or lie flat. The giver lies over their partner's back, with legs on the outside and supporting themselves with their hands.

What's Good About It

It's a chill, lazy position that's great for morning wake-up sex; slow, languorous weekend sex; or sleepy "I love you" nighttime sex.

Tweak It

Go for maximum cuddliness by having the giver brace themselves up on their arms to kiss and nibble on their partner's cheeks, eyes, ears, and neck. Try gentle nips, licks, and sucks. The receiver can lift themselves on their forearms and expose more of their neck and shoulders to get even more.

Make It Even Better

Put the focus on the receiver's pleasure by putting a pillow under their hips and propping a vibe on it—anything from a small bullet vibe to a big industrial strength wand vibrator will work. The giver can whisper sweet or filthy things into the receiver's ear, tell them how amazing they feel, or concoct a full-on sexy story to tell them as they slowly pump into them.

49 The Congress of the Elephant

Congress is in session.

How to Do It

The receiver lies on their stomach, pressing their head, chest, and arms into the bed, with their hips slightly lifted. The giver lies over their partner to enter from behind. The giver holds their weight on their hands and knees—their chest is touching the partner's back, not crushing it.

What's Good About It

This provides lots of closeness and is great for larger penises or strap-ons, whether it's anally or vaginally.

Tweak It

The receiver can prop their hips up on a pillow or sex wedge and lie on their hand. If they have a vulva, they can rub two fingers along each side of their clit or hump their lubed-up fingers or the palm of their hand. If they have a penis, they can rub the bottom of their shaft with a lubed hand or fill their hand with lube and make a tunnel to wrap around their penis.

Make It Even Better

This is a great segue from a long, sexy massage. The giver can start making the massage a little more X-rated, bit by bit, rubbing their hands up their partner's inner thigh and teasing them by brushing against their vulva or penis. When the receiver starts arching their back for more, make 'em wait a little longer, then go on it.

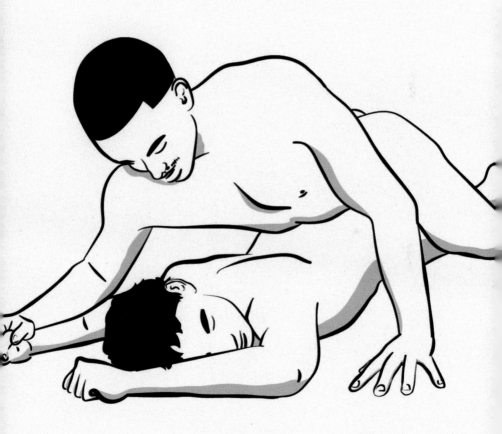

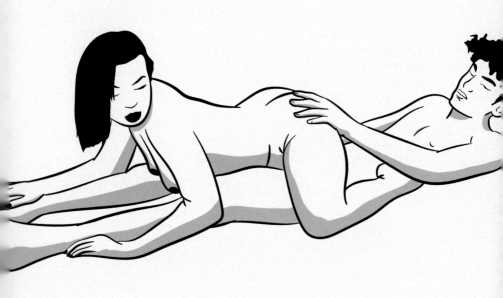

50

Inversion

Horizontal twerking.

How to Do It

The giver lies on their back with the receiver crouching over them and facing away. The receiver holds themselves on their hand and knee and slides their partner's penis or strap-on inside them. The receiver's hands rest on either side of their partner's legs and their legs are wrapped against the partner's thighs for support.

What's Good About It

This is a great position for the person on top to control the movement. They can roll their hips, rock back and forth, grind or move up and down to thrust. Also good for receivers who like to show off dat ass and/or givers who like to look at said ass.

Tweak It

Holding onto each other's feet and stroking them as you move together feels surprisingly grounding and connected. Try lacing your fingers between each other's toes.

Make It Even Better

Play up the butt-centric nature of Inversion. The giver can squeeze, pull, knead, pinch, slap, or spank those cheeks. If the receiver is into it, the giver can use a paddle or whip across the backside or slide fingers or a sex toy inside. The receiver can tease their partner by rolling and gyrating their hips.

51

One Knot

Ready, set, gooooooo.

How to Do It

The giver kneels on the bed. The receiver squats back onto the giver's lap, then bends over so their chest is pushed against their thighs.

What's Good About It

If you two want sex that feels really raw and immediate, this is it.

Tweak It

This takes some balance (and iron-strong thigh muscles). For support, the receiver can press their hands to the bed or hold onto a sturdy headboard. The giver can help out by holding onto their partner's hips or thighs. You can also try it on the bottom steps of a staircase, with the giver kneeling a few steps lower than the receiver.

Make It Even Better

Foreplay makes everything better. No one magically knows what their partner likes, so you get to learn about each other. You can just start touching your partner and get feedback as you go along. You can use actual words like "over to the side a bit more" or "faster" or just convey what's working via moans. You can also masturbate in front of each other to see how your partner touches themselves. Or you can put your hand on top of your partner's hand on your penis or vulva and guide them.

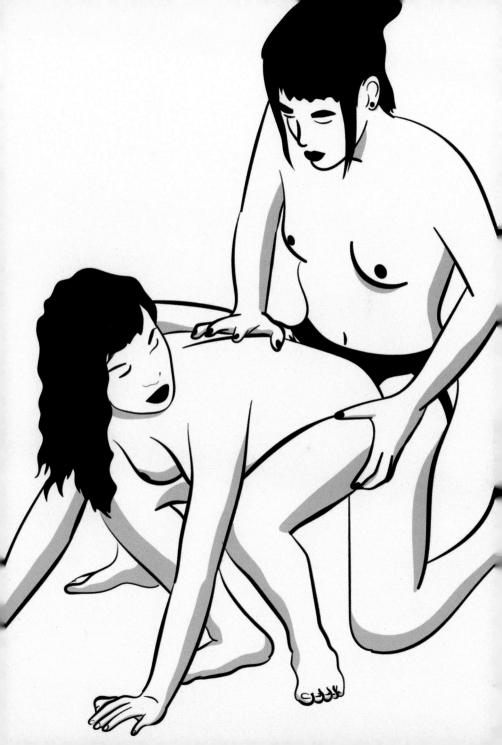

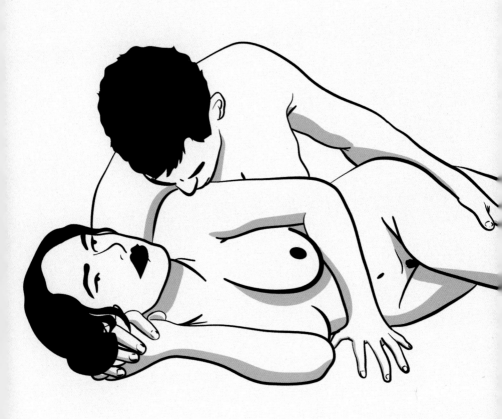

52

The Rhino

Good ol' spooning, Kama Sutra–style.

How to Do It

The receiver lies on their side. The giver lies behind them, wrapping their arms around their partner.

What's Good About It

Full body contact, and everyone gets to lie down. It's like hugging and having sex at the same time.

Tweak It

Give the receiver more stimulation in front with a reach around. The giver can play with their partner's penis or vulva, matching their hand motions to the thrusts. If the little spoon has a larger-sized body, try a long-handled vibrator like a wand for easier access.

Make It Even Better

Try the Rhino for sleepy all-night sex. At bedtime, get each other close to orgasm, but don't let each other finish yet. Go to sleep in each other's arms, midpenetration or with the big spoon's hand cupping little spoon's groin. Boners will go soft, you'll shift positions and such, but whenever one of you wakes up, share some sleepy kisses, a few lazy thrusts, some loving strokes to each other's penis or vulva, or just press against your partner. Spend the whole night in sleepy lusty bliss. When you wake up, you will be beyond ready for each other.

THE POSITIONS

53

The Rear-Entry Stride

Hoo-boy. You been doing those stretches?

How to Do It

The giver stands with their legs spread and feet firmly on the ground. The receiver gets on their hands and knees in front of the giver, facing away. The giver lifts one of the receiver's ankles and puts it on their shoulder. The receiver is holding themselves up on their hands like they're doing a handstand.

What's Good About It

This is an amped up version of doggie with an even better view for the giver. The giver can watch themselves sliding into their partner while getting an excellent view of their partner's ass.

Tweak It

The average person is probably not going to be able to do this *exactly* as it's illustrated. Totally fine! The receiver can try spreading their legs wider and bending them slightly, or just use a chair, cushions, or even the side of the bed to prop themselves up.

Make It Even Better

With no eye contact and little skin-to-skin touching, this position doesn't seem like it would be an intimate position, but the intimacy comes through in other ways. Since you can't see each other, you need to work together to communicate what you want. Let each other know what you need via touch and sound.

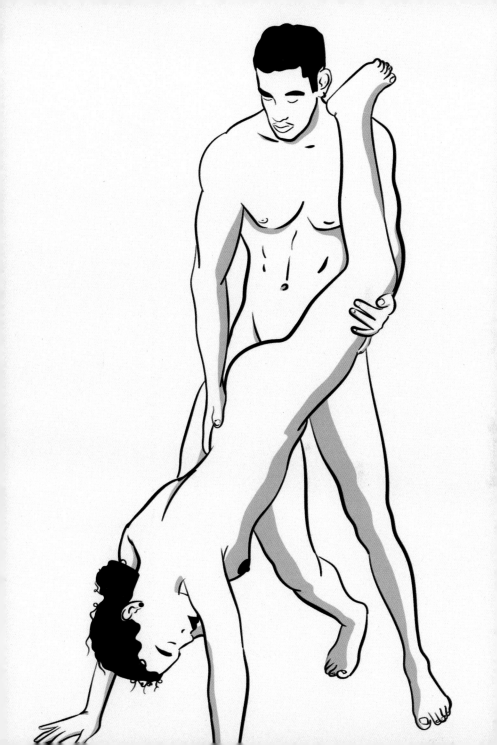

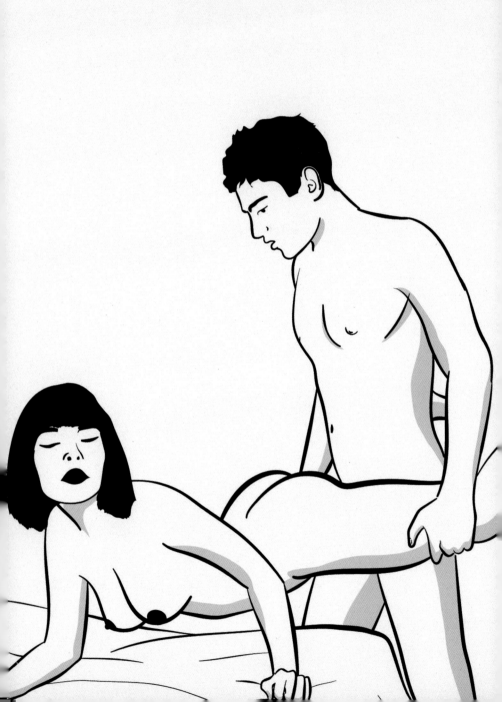

54 The Thunderbolt or the Wheelbarrow

Like a company picnic game, but naked and with sex.

How to Do It

The receiver lies on the bed face down. The giver stands at the edge of the bed or kneels on the bed. They lift the receiver's legs with their hands, like the old wheelbarrow game.

What's Good About It

Besides being ready in case a game of naked wheelbarrow racing breaks out, this position allows the giver to use lots of different types of thrusting—quick and shallow, deep and fast, or pressing close and grinding. To switch it up even more, the giver can raise or lower the receiver's legs or open and close them like a pair of hedge clippers.

Tweak It

This isn't exactly inherently comfortable, so figure out ways to make it so. The receiver can try it on their hands or resting on their forearms. If that's not working, try a stack of firm pillows or some sofa cushions. If the giver doesn't have super strength, the receiver can carry more of their own weight on their arms and pillows. You'll figure it out.

Make It Even Better

This wheelbarrow can travel. Turn it into a competitive event by trying it in every room of the home. It can work on a bed, couch, table, desk, counter, or set of stairs.

55

The Wrestler

Getting pinned.

How to Do It

The receiver lies on their belly and bends their legs, getting their feet as close as possible to their butt and holding their feet by their ankles. The giver kneels between their partner's legs, lifting their partner's legs off the bed and pulling their partner close to enter.

What's Good About It

This has opportunities for ass play and is good for experimenting with BDSM scenarios with spanking, dominance, and submission or bondage.

Tweak It

To get into the position, the giver can help by holding their partner's legs in position, making sure to get feedback so they don't overbend them. Use pillows under the receiver to tilt their pelvis and allow easier penetration. And as always, if body parts aren't cooperating, abandon ship and find a way that works for you both.

Make It Even Better

Experimenting with sensation play keeps the receiver in a state of high arousal and anticipation. Run things like a leather belt, a feather, or a silky scarf over the receiver's butt cheeks, back, and legs. The giver can also try cold versus heat by running an ice cube down the partner's thigh coupled with a dollop of warming lube dripping down their ass crack.

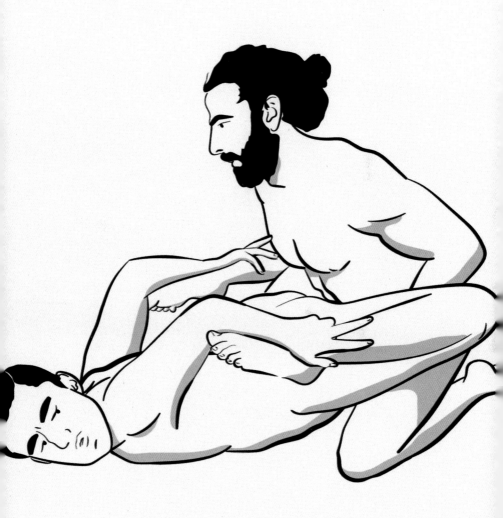

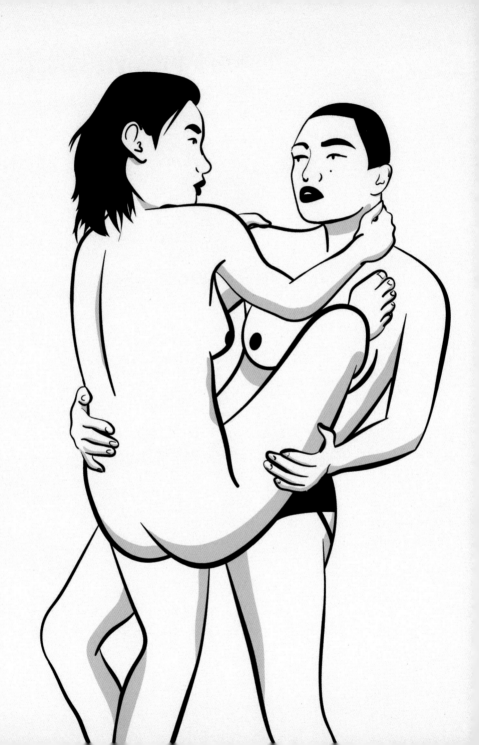

56

The Encircling

Scratch that.

How to Do It

The giver stands against a wall. The receiver stands and faces their partner, putting one foot against the giver's heart. The giver holds their partner closely to give them support.

What's Good About It

The position puts you in a combative stance. Go ahead and play with that.

Tweak It

Try a little braggy trash talk. Don't be mean, obviously, unless you're into that, but tell each other what you're going to do with them or how hard you're gonna make them cum.

Make It Even Better

Ready to go into full battle mode? The Kama Sutra recommends scratching "when love becomes intense." The text recommends eight different types of scratches to be used when y'all are full of passion. That you? You can lightly scratch your partner's neck, thighs, chest, or arms, run your fingernails down each other's backs, or dig those nails in when orgasm is nigh. Want OG advice from the original text? Try one of these: "The curved mark with the nails, which is impressed on the neck and the breasts, is called the 'half moon.'" Or "When five marks with the nails are made close to one another near the nipple of the breast, it is called 'the jump of a hare.'"

57 The Face-to-Face Position

Bite me.

How to Do It

The receiver stands with their back against a wall with their legs spread. The giver stands to enter, holding their partner's hands against the wall. The receiver circles their hips to provide the movement, or the giver can thrust away.

What's Good About It

This is all about the drama, less about taking a straight path to orgasm.

Tweak It

If the receiver fantasizes about being ravished or taken, the giver can play into it by pinning their partner's hands against the wall and aggressively kissing them while they penetrate.

Make It Even Better

Go even harder with the theatrics by adding biting. (With all the consent, of course.) The Kama Sutra describes several types of bites. If you both are down for it, try Discrete (biting of the lower lip), Coral Jewel (marks left when the same spot is squeezed several times between the top teeth and lower lip), or Scattered Clouds (circle of small, irregular toothmarks beneath the breasts). If you like the idea of biting without the actual biting, try some toothless neck nibbling for some in-home vampire fan fic. "All the places that can be kissed, are also the places that can be bitten, except the upper lip, the interior of the mouth, and the eyes," reads the Kama Sutra. So no biting anyone's eyes.

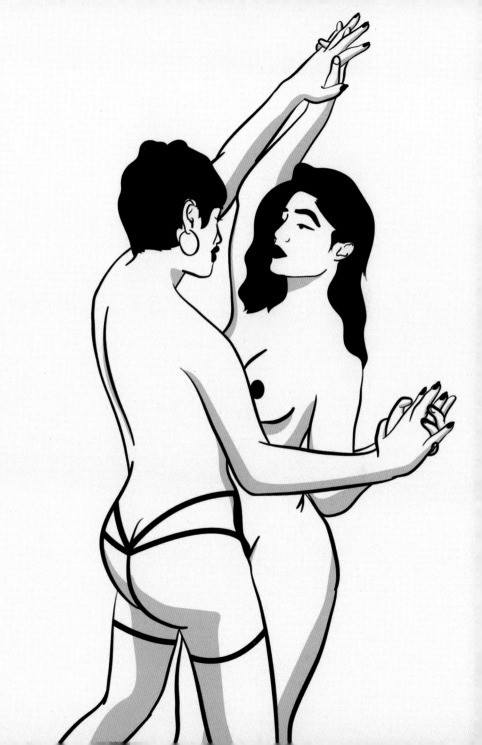

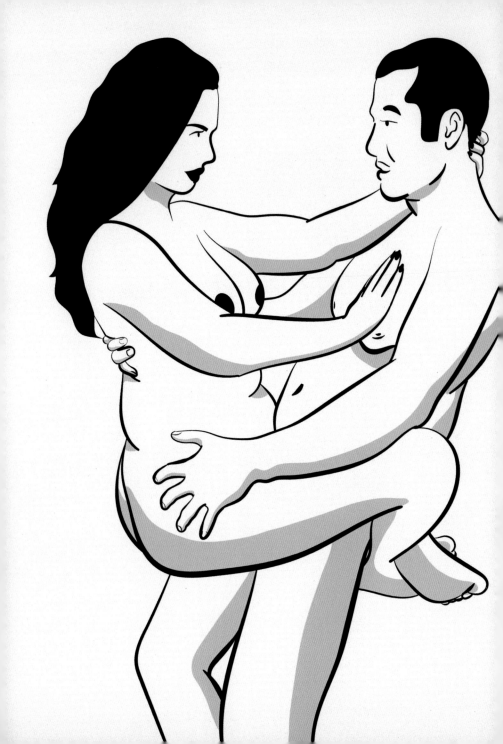

58

Fame

Up you go.

How to Do It

The giver stands, feet hip-distance apart, and braces themselves with their legs. They can either lift the receiver onto their penis or strap-on, or the receiver can jump up into their arms. The receiver wraps their legs around the giver's waist to stay put.

What's Good About It

Lots of eye contact so you can gaze at each other to celebrate your accomplishment in doing it.

Tweak It

Try this when you're taking the action from the couch to the bedroom and don't want to be apart for even a second. It's part sexy, part just fun.

Make It Even Better

The giver can blindfold the receiver and carry them to a room that they've set up beforehand. Go ahead and set a theme for the evening. Go full dungeon mode with an array of gear laid out on the bed like handcuffs, floggers, and fetish clothing. Or prep for romance novel sex with soft music, rose petals on the bed, scented candles, and a bottle of champagne chilling at the bedside. Or maybe try sex playroom and set up the night table with a selection of toys for both of you, edible lube, and this book open to a particular page.

59 The Knee–Elbow Position

G-whiz.

How to Do It

Both people stand facing each other. The giver braces themselves with their legs and lifts the receiver, holding them up by their butt. The giver uses the crook of their elbow to hold their partner by the knees, and the receiver wraps their arms around their partner's neck.

What's Good About It

This is great for allowing the giver to completely control the movement by moving the receiver's butt up and down over their penis or strap-on. It's not a super sustainable position for most people, so use it as a transition position for moving the action from one room to another in dramatic fashion.

Tweak It

Have the giver stand with their back against the wall for more support.

Make It Even Better

This is great for G-spot and P-spot stimulation, but if you want more intense stimulation, take the pose to your bed so the giver can use their hands. For both G- and P-spots, the technique is similar. The giver slides a lubed finger inside their partner's vagina or butt and presses, rubs, or taps on the upper wall, about an inch or two inside. Some women with vulvas can squirt with intense G-spot and clitoral stimulation, so throw down some towels first.

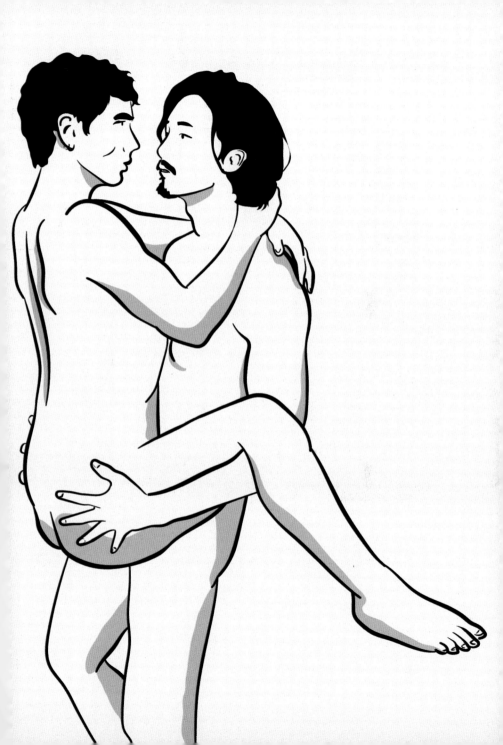

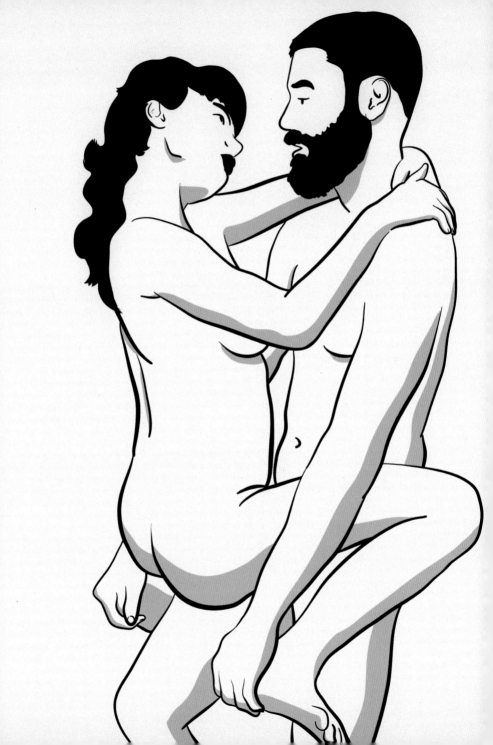

60

Two Palms

You are so in for it.

How to Do It

The giver stands against a wall. The receiver hops up on their partner's body, clamping their thighs around the giver's hips and clinging to their neck. The giver holds onto each of their partner's feet with their hands.

What's Good About It

This is a twist on standing positions because the receiver is controlling the motion by pushing themselves up and down on their partner's penis or strap-on while looking into their eyes.

Tweak It

If you two like the feel of this but can't maintain the position, have the giver sit their butt on the edge of a counter, table, or sturdy barstool.

Make It Even Better

The Kama Sutra has a whole section on hitting, including types of blows, where to hit, and the sounds to make when being struck. If you want to explore this a bit, you'll need to set some ground rules first. Choose a safe word, decide what will happen, and communicate throughout. You can use an open hand or go fancier and invest in a paddle or flogger. If you want to DIY it, you can use a ruler, hairbrush, or table tennis paddle.

61 The Standing Stride

Hit the showers.

How to Do It

The giver stands, feet hip-distance apart, and braces themselves with their legs. The receiver stands facing their partner and lifts a leg for easier penetration. Both people wrap their arms around each other for balance.

What's Good About It

This is a good standing position if no one wants to be carrying anyone else (valid). The receiver just puts their leg up and, bam, you're go to go.

Tweak It

If there's a big height difference, you can bend your knees to get parts lined up, or the shorter person can stand on a sturdy step stool.

Make It Even Better

This is the rare position that actually works in the shower, but you need to be super safe. Create a fall-free area by putting down a sexy nonskid floor mat and making sure there are sturdy things to hold onto like grab bars. Use a silicone lube that will last under water. And, in nonsafety news, a detachable showerhead is a stellar way to make a vulva happy. Use it as an enhancement for penetrative sex or just on its own. Just get the water to a comfortable temp, point, and shoot.

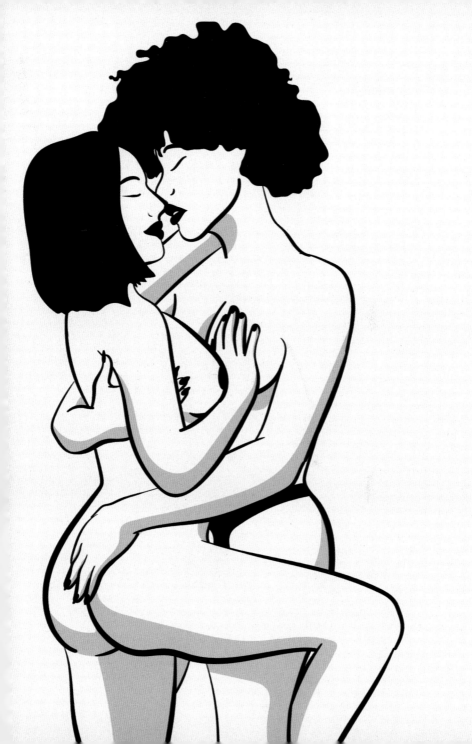

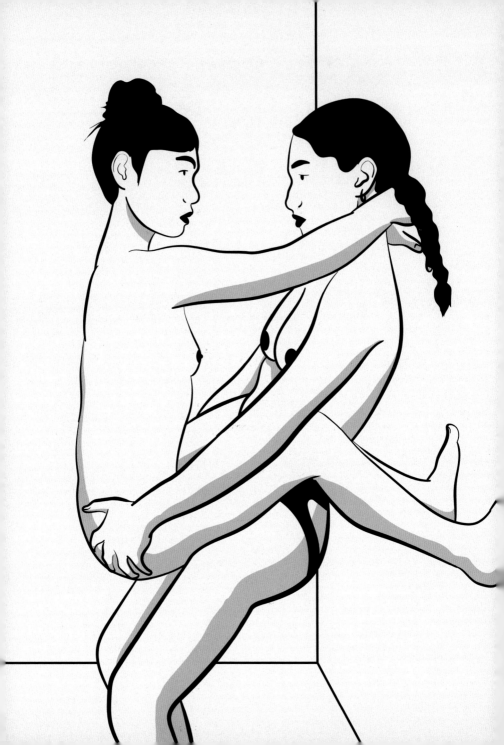

62 The Suspended Position

Get up against the wall.

How to Do It

The giver stands next to a wall with their legs apart and knees bent. They cradle the receiver's butt in their arms and hold them against their penis or strap-on, leaning back for more leverage. The receiver wraps their arms around their partner's neck and legs around their waist, using their thighs to hold on. The receiver presses their feet against the wall for stability and to control the motion.

What's Good About It

It has all the "take me now" vibes of a standing position but offers more stability than most standing positions because both people can make use of the wall for support.

Tweak It

Sharing your fantasies can be incredibly hot. Try whispering a fantasy in your partner's ear while you're moving together. (If you are fantasizing about someone else, the Kama Sutra is down with that too. It's called the "congress of transferred love." Maybe don't share that one though.)

Make It Even Better

Keep a standing position going for much longer by investing in a sex swing. They'll keep you in position but don't require the feats of strength. There are simple ones that hang from a doorjamb or more intricate versions with a padded seat.

THE POSITIONS

63 The Standing Swing

Get carried away.

How to Do It

The giver stands with their back against a wall or doorjamb with knees flexed for support. The receiver wraps their arms around their partner's neck and circles their legs around the giver's hips, keeping themselves steady by wrapping their feet behind the partner's knees.

What's Good About It

Lots of face-to-face contact, plus the general swooniness of one of you carrying the other like a sexy firefighter.

Tweak It

This is hard to maintain, so use it as a transport position to passionately take your L-O-V-E to a more comfortable room. If you dig the feel of the position but the giver's arms are starting to shake, do it next to a counter so that the giver can hoist the receiver onto the edge of a counter-top or barstool and keep it going.

Make It Even Better

Harness the weightlessness of taking this position underwater. The lifting that was difficult-to-impossible on dry land suddenly becomes easy when you're in a pool. To avoid getting arrested for indecent exposure (and bein' too sexy), you'll need a private pool where you won't be interrupted. And make sure you use silicone lube to keep everything slippery because water is an anti-lube that, weirdly, makes everything drier.

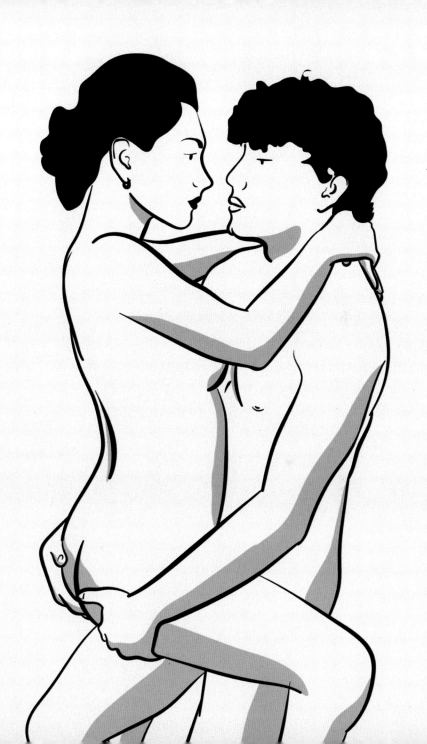

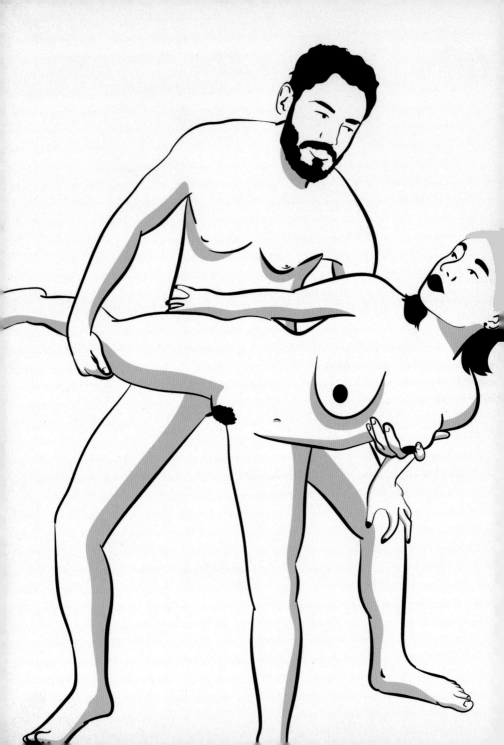

64

The Tripod

Strike a pose.

How to Do It

The giver stands behind their partner. They lift one of the receiver's knees into the air, holding them by the knee. The giver supports their partner with the other hand, either holding onto their thigh, their waists, or their chest. The receiver has their leg as straight as possible behind them.

What's Good About It

The giver has wide leeway for thrusting, and both people have a free hand to stroke the receiver. Plus y'all just look epic.

Tweak It

It can be super hot to watch yourselves in a mirror. And this is especially good for it because you're looking so good. Angle yourself so you highlight whatever turns you on, whether it's watching your faces, a bouncing pair of boobs, or a rear view.

Make It Even Better

Is using toys consistent with the Kama Sutra? Yes! It didn't exactly mention ten-speed wand vibrators, but it does talk about using dildos to enhance the experience. In honor of those early sex toys, try adding a dildo to the Tripod. Use a dildo on a penis-having partner for a different anal experience, or if the receiver has a vulva, add a dildo for double penetration.